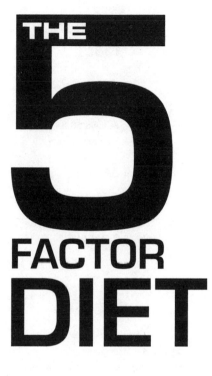

THE 5 FACTOR DIET

Meredith® Books
Des Moines, Iowa

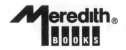

Meredith Books
1716 Locust Street
Des Moines, Iowa 50309-3023
meredithbooks.com

Printed in the United States of America.

First Edition.
Library of Congress Control Number: 2006930029
ISBN-13: 978-0-696-23224-4

See your doctor first.
This diet and fitness book is designed to provide helpful information on the subjects addressed.
This book is sold with the understanding that the author and publisher are not rendering
medical, health, or other personal services. The suggestions for specific exercise routines,
foods, and lifestyle recommendations are not intended to replace medical advice or treatment
by your physician. All questions and concerns regarding your health, metabolism, weight,
nutrition, and physical activity should be directed to your physician, particularly if you have
any health problems or medical problems (including if you are pregnant or lactating). All
reasonable attempts have been made to include the most recent and factual research and
medical reports regarding exercise and nutrition. However, there is no guarantee that future
research, particularly human studies, will not change the information presented here. Individual
needs vary, and no nutrition or exercise program will meet everyone's needs. Be sure to consult
your physician prior to following any of the suggestions presented in this book and also before
changing your diet or exercise routine. You should rely on your physician's advice regarding
whether the suggestions presented in this book are appropriate for you and you should rely
on your physician to establish your weight goal. The author and publisher disclaim all liability
associated with the recommendations and guidelines set forth in this book. Further, the Internet
addresses in this book were accurate at the time of printing.

This book is dedicated to all my clients.
You have been, and continue to be, my
guinea pigs, my inspiration, and my friends.

ACKNOWLEDGMENTS

My parents. To whom I owe all my success.

My brothers, Jesse and Bobby. My best friends and my fountain of youth.

My manager, Kristin Giese. I treasure your leadership and strength.

My literary agent, Andrea Barzvi. The only agent I will ever have.

My cowriter, Myatt Murphy. For sharing my vision and being so professional.

My editor, Stephanie Karpinske. For polishing the words.

Paola Patrella. For your delicious recipes.

Logan Alexander. For your photography and humor.

Carmen Bonicci. My Canadian strategist.

My commercial agent, Brittany Balbo, for your support.

My closest friends, Dave, Anne, Behzad, Sam, Rachel, Wendy, Michael, David, Jamie, Ricky, Jeff, Josh, David, Rick, John, Brian, Jen, Jodi, Vera, and Wil. For reminding me where I'm from and who I am.

Lucy and Viv. You are always in my heart.

Contents

This book took me 15 years to write.

Not really 15 years of writing ... more like a decade and a half of evolution.

The 5-Factor evolution started when I was a "husky" teenager ("husky" is simply a kinder way of saying overweight). I bought every diet book, fitness magazine, and exotic weight loss pill, powder, and bar! I tried weight training, step aerobics classes, Pilates, and yoga. I experimented with diets such as Pritikin, Body For Life, and the Zone. I became interested in exercise and nutrition as a way to make me look and feel better. However, it wasn't until both of my younger brothers were diagnosed with type 1 diabetes that I became interested in the science of food and how it affects our bodies. I spent eight years in university studying metabolism, biochemistry, nutrition, and physiology. I call this period my "nerd years."

While I was in graduate school, the 5-Factor evolution continued as I began to work as a nutrition scientist for the Canadian Department of National Defense. I learned a great deal about research. Not only did I perform my own nutrition studies (breaking many test tubes in the process), but I also learned how to assess existing nutrition research. Equipped with studies that could definitively support or refute popular diet info, I began to question many dietary practices. I thought more critically about claims I heard about popular diet programs and weight loss supplements.

I reread all the diet books I had previously treated as gospel and underlined all of the "facts" the books used to support their claims. I then set out to find the research these claims were based on. To my chagrin, I realized most diets and weight loss strategies are quick-fix programs based on half-truths and flat-out fabrications.

I knew there had to be a way of eating healthy that would also be realistic. I wanted a program based on real truth, real science, and real people's lifestyles, a sensible system that would promote fat loss *and* enjoyment.

My 5-Factor evolution continued as my nutrition and fitness practice grew. I developed and refined my nutrition plan and applied it to clients with amazing results. My program garnered the attention of actors who wanted to tone up for upcoming roles. Nineteen films, nine television shows, and more than 50 actor and musician clients later, my 5-Factor Diet has helped the likes of Halle Berry, Alicia Keys, Kanye West, Mandy Moore, Eva Mendes, Rachel Weisz, Rick Fox, John Mayer, Brendan Fraser, Stephen Dorff, Robert Downey Jr., and Benjamin Bratt.

In 2005 my first book, *5-Factor Fitness*, hit the top of two bestseller lists. Though *5-Factor Fitness* was primarily an exercise plan, it contained a brief introduction to the 5-Factor Diet and offered a number of quick 5-Factor recipes. I received more than 5,000 emails from people who had purchased *5-Factor Fitness* and had shed anywhere from 5 to 87 pounds! Nearly all of them requested more 5-Factor recipes and wanted to know more about the 5-Factor Diet.

So, with great pride, I present you with the last diet book you will ever purchase. Welcome to *The 5-Factor Diet*.

Harley Pasternak, M.Sc.

CHAPTER 1

A Fresh Start

We've met before.

I don't know your name or where you live, but it's safe to say that I do know you—and I know why you're reading this book.

You're not happy with your body.

It doesn't matter whether you're looking to drop a few pounds, firm up, or improve your health so you can live a longer life; all of these goals start with eating right.

Most likely you've already tried some—it probably seems like *all*—of the different diets that are popular today. It's likely that you even lost some weight. But if you're like most people, you gained some or all of it back. Or worse, you regained it all plus a few extra pounds. You're sick and tired of fighting the "fat war," running caloric calculations in your head and denying yourself entire food groups. You're fed up with weighing your food at every meal, scrimping on portions, and eating tasteless diet foods while salivating over the cooking shows on TV—all in an effort to look as lean, fit, and glamorous as the movie stars you admire on the big screen.

Well, I have some news for you. Television actors and movie stars don't make the same mistakes that you have. And with the 5-Factor Diet, you won't make those mistakes ever again. Absolutely anyone can get into better shape quickly—the harder part, of course, is staying that way. 5-Factor can help.

MY HOLLYWOOD SECRETS ARE NOW YOURS

When my first book, 5-Factor Fitness, became an overnight success in 2005, I was proud that the system I've been using for years with my Hollywood clients was finally available to everyone. In the book I outlined a 5-week program to jump-start readers to a better body and healthier lifestyle, focusing primarily on fitness and exercise.

Since the book was published, I've been overwhelmed with requests from readers like you asking for more information on diet and nutrition. The sheer volume of letters I've received has made it clear to me that people want to know more about the nutritional plan I use with my clients—particularly the 5-minute meals that are part of my program—and how to incorporate it into their day-to-day lives.

The 5-Factor Diet book you're holding is my new nutritional bible, a complete guide to the simple yet extraordinarily effective diet program I've used for years with my celebrity clients to get them—and keep them—in great shape.

My 5-Factor Diet stands alone as a nutritional program that is simple yet comprehensive. More important, it actually works. Having this book on your shelf will be like having your very own round-the-clock personal nutritionist and chef on hand. It's the result of my many years of education and experience in the weight loss industry, with proven results you can see anytime one of my celebrity clients makes a movie, strolls down the red carpet, or poses for a magazine. The 5-Factor Diet is not just another diet book. I promise, this will be the last diet book you'll ever need.

THE 5-FACTOR DIET

So why do I call my program the 5-Factor Diet? That's easy! Or, I should say, it's to make things easier for you. Every nutritional and

> "I suffered from extremely poor health and almost died twice within the same year, a situation that left me too sick and unable to exercise for over three years. I had no energy and I gave up exercise altogether until I tried 5-Factor. The simplicity of the plan and, more important, seeing amazingly quick results made it easy for me to stay dedicated to the program. It's magic!"
>
> **Louise Meinardus** AGE: **40s** WEIGHT LOST SO FAR: **5 lbs.**

exercise principle I'm about to teach you breaks down into five easy-to-remember points:

+ The 5-Factor Diet is a 5-week diet plan.
+ There are 5 types of food you should eat in every meal.
+ The Diet incorporates a 5-phase 5-Factor Hollywood Workout.
+ My exercise routine, like my diet, is simple: 5 workouts a week, each consisting of five 5-minute phases.
+ To follow my diet, you'll want to try some of my 100-plus 5-Factor recipes, which require only 5 (or fewer) main ingredients. Each delicious recipe can be prepared in 5 minutes or less. (That doesn't count cooking time, of course; I said delicious, not miraculous!)

I promise: If you can count to 5, the 5-Factor Diet will be the easiest diet you'll ever use to lose.

YOU'RE READY TO START!

Before I get into detail about the simplicity and effectiveness of the 5-Factor Diet—and teach you the scientific basis for it—I want to talk to you about all the fad diets you may have tried in the past. Because you can't move forward without figuring out why you've been falling

backward, it's important to understand why every other diet has ultimately failed you. Turn the page to finally break yourself of the yo-yo
diet cycle forever.

Sophia Bush ACTRESS, STAR OF THE TV HIT *ONE TREE HILL*

---

*"To me, Harley's plan is an eating and fitness
plan that makes sense, allows me to eat
real food, and gives me compact, effective
workouts. I actually crave a healthy lifestyle.
It feels incredible!"*

CHAPTER 2

Fad Diets Don't Work

A client came to me about 40 pounds overweight and frustrated. Over the three preceding years, he had lost 200 pounds, desperately trying a variety of fad diets. Sounds impressive, right?

It wasn't.

When I say he lost 200 pounds, that's counting the weight he had lost and gained back. He would drop 40 pounds, then gain 50 back. He would lose 50 pounds, then gain 60 back! It's called yo-yo dieting or weight cycling. It's not just a waste of your time; it could do your body harm.

Today's fad diets are merely the latest in a long line of ineffective and often dangerous diet crazes. Over the past 20 years, Americans have been bombarded with one diet after another. Though the diets appear to be as different from each other as night and day, they all have something in common: They only work *up to a certain point*, if they work at all.

I believe that once you understand why these diets fall short, you can choose a more sensible plan and achieve the body and healthy lifestyle you've always hoped for. I don't want you to waste any more time or effort on diets that won't work. Failure is something your body simply can't afford.

In doing research for the 5-Factor Diet, I read dozens of diet books. As someone who makes a living educating people about health and fitness, I was shocked at how ridiculous many of these diets were.

You see, whenever you begin a low-calorie diet, your body notices that it's being fed fewer calories and immediately lowers your basal metabolic rate (BMR)—the rate at which your body burns calories. That means the result of eating fewer calories is burning fewer calories all day long. Once you quit the diet—and you will—it takes a while for your body to bring your BMR back to normal.

That's why yo-yo dieters end up gaining more and more weight with each diet failure. If you go back to your old eating habits while your BMR is still low, you won't just regain the pounds you lost, you'll pack a few extra on top. Repeat this cycle a few times and you end up gaining more weight the more often you try to lose it. It's physically exhausting and emotionally frustrating.

I want you to ask yourself what I consider the single most important health and fitness question: Do you want to look good tomorrow or do you want to look good for the rest of your life?

You need to think of your health and fitness goals as a marathon instead of a sprint. Most fad diets claim they can help you drop pounds fast, and I know that promise can be incredibly alluring. But that weight loss is usually the result of nutritional tactics that are not only unhealthy but also impossible to maintain.

To take pounds off for good, it's all about finishing the race. You need an effective and efficient plan of attack that lets you lose weight consistently, not just immediately. What differentiates the 5-Factor Diet from all the fad diets that I'm about to discuss is this: While all of these fad diets work for a short time, only the 5-Factor Diet will keep you lean and healthy for a lifetime.

BLOOD TYPE DIET

This diet claims it's your blood type, not just the calories you consume, that causes weight gain. According to the program, the secret to losing fat is to eat only specific foods that are compatible with your blood type. Eating the wrong foods is supposedly like receiving a transfusion of the wrong type of blood, causing substances from your food, called lectins, to enter your bloodstream. It's this flow of lectins that supposedly causes blood cells to clot, leading to a variety of health issues.

The diet's claims about blood type and weight loss are not backed up by relevant scientific research. Your blood type has nothing to do with your body's ability to burn excess fat. The plan restricts not only calories but food types as well. You're told not to eat certain healthy foods that are rich in antioxidants, vitamins, and minerals. And the diet recommends some unusual foods and supplements that are only available online.

CABBAGE SOUP DIET

It's easy to see why so many people have tried this strict, low-calorie program that has been around for decades. Its proponents claim you can drop up to 20 pounds in seven days by eating little more than cabbage-based soup several times a day. Cycling on and off the diet (7 days on, 14 days off) is said to promote rapid weight loss.

This diet can be harmful to your body because it restricts your caloric intake to less than 1,000 calories a day. It leaves you feeling perpetually hungry because you're basically forcing your body to live off nothing but fiber and water. There's no protein or fats and few vitamins or minerals. The weight loss most people see is almost always water and lean muscle mass because the lack of protein causes your body to cannibalize its own muscle tissue. You will also likely have uncomfortable side effects such as diarrhea, abdominal pain, light-headedness, and flatulence.

GRAPEFRUIT DIET

In this popular diet, you're required to eat a whole grapefruit with every meal. Why a grapefruit? According to the diet, grapefruits contain a special fat-burning enzyme.

The negatives of this diet are identical to those of the Cabbage Soup Diet, even though the plan does allow small amounts of protein. It's not the grapefruit that deserves the credit for whatever weight is lost; this restrictive, 800-calorie diet basically starves you. No matter how much you may wish otherwise, there is simply no such thing as a superfood with magical abilities to make you lose weight.

CAVEMAN DIET

The creators of this nutrition plan believe that cavemen and cavewomen were lean and healthy because of the all-natural foods they ate. According to this diet, processed and cultivated foods, including wheat and grains, are the true cause of all major disease and obesity. The diet requires you to return to your Neanderthal roots by eating only what your ancestors did. That means eliminating all processed foods in favor of natural foods such as fish, lean meats, berries, vegetables, fruits, nuts, and seeds.

I can't argue with the premise that the less processed a food is, the healthier it is for your body. However, it is a stretch to claim that the lack of processed foods was the main reason our ancestors were leaner than we are. But they also had to spend many physically demanding hours hunting down or picking their own food.

Cavemen were so lean in part because they were much more physically active than we are today. Yet that factor is never considered in the caveman equation. Nor does the diet discuss the fact that our ancestors lacked convenient access to food and thus ate significantly less than we do. And there is no scientific research to date that links wheat or grains to obesity and resulting diseases—yet this diet claims that corn is responsible for more cancer deaths than cigarettes. There is a more logical reason why our ancestors didn't suffer from cancer, heart disease, and other

"I tried practically every fad diet invented, but they never worked long term. The 5-Factor Diet opened my eyes to correct, healthy eating. By following Harley's plan, I was finally able to learn to change my eating habits. Diets come and go, but Harley's plan is for the rest of your life!"

Danielle Martin AGE: **37** WEIGHT LOST SO FAR: **77 lbs.**

Sanaa Lathan ACTRESS AND STAR OF THE MOVIE *LOVE AND BASKETBALL*

"I was asked to lose some weight for my last film. Harley had me do his 5-Factor Diet and exercise program. Within weeks my body was transformed. Getting in shape was never this easy. And I just saw my movie. And if I may say so myself, my body looks better than it ever has on film. I'm a fan for life."

modern-day ailments: They never grew old because the average life span of a Neanderthal man was 20 years!

NO SUGAR DIET
This diet eliminates foods that are high in refined sugar and carbohydrates that rank high on the glycemic index.

Break out your calculator because you'll have to make sure every meal is divided into 30 percent carbohydrates, 30 percent protein, and 40 percent fat. Not only are these calculations time-consuming, but your daily caloric consumption is limited to an unhealthy 1,200 calories. You don't lose weight because you're eating less sugar; you lose it because you're eating too few calories. The diet restricts many healthy-for-you foods, such as carrots, that contain ample amounts of essential vitamins and minerals. Instead, it claims you can lose weight while eating high-fat, low-sugar foods such as hamburger, steak, and cheese.

LIQUID DIETS
These diets make you forgo food in favor of a liquid meal replacement drink typically made from sugar, fat-free milk powder, fiber, vitamins, and

minerals. On some versions of the plan you eat only shakes; on others you also have small, low-calorie meals.

One of my clients was on a shake diet for a while. Every day she drank five shakes instead of eating real food. She was miserable and depressed, especially when she went out to dinner at a five-star restaurant and had to bring a shake with her instead of eating the delicious meals.

Liquid diets are antisocial, and they're not sustainable because they're not satisfying. Research has shown that liquids don't fill your stomach as effectively as solid foods. And most of these shakes are deficient in dietary fiber, so you never feel quite as full. These low-calorie diets—as low as 700 calories—can stress your kidneys because many liquid dieters end up dehydrated.

NEW BEVERLY HILLS DIET

This diet has you combine foods in particular ways in order to create a certain mix of enzymes that supposedly helps your body properly digest your food.

Although combining certain types of foods can be beneficial for losing weight—something I'll explain later as part of the 5-Factor Diet—but it's not because of the enyme mix in food, as this diet claims. The truth is, the enzymes used to digest food are created by your body.

The theory that any food that can't be digested properly "adds" weight doesn't make sense either. If your body can't break down food, that means it has less chance to grab the calories and store them as body fat. Regardless of theories, this diet is also too low in protein, vitamins, and minerals to be considered healthy.

BODY FOR LIFE

This is a six-day-a-week diet and exercise plan whose creator promises that you'll be in the best shape of your life after 12 weeks.

You'll notice that Body For Life encourages you to use a lot of nutritional supplements. In fact, the program seems to be designed mainly to sell these supplements. One thing I do approve of about the Body For Life plan is that it encourages regular exercise.

HIGH-FIBER DIETS

The theory behind super-high-fiber diets is that if you overeat fibrous foods, your meals travel through your digestive system at an accelerated

"**Your book turned my life around after 15 years away from the gym had taken its toll. It was exactly what I needed to get back on track! I started using 5-Factor when I weighed 250 pounds and had a 42-inch waist. I am currently 185 pounds with a 32-inch waist. I feel amazing! Your book has given me the desire and discipline to attain a physical goal I thought was part of my past and never to be seen again!**"

Andrew White AGE: **39** WEIGHT LOST SO FAR: **65 lbs.**

pace, preventing your body from absorbing all the calories.

Eating fiber daily offers many health benefits. But eating excessive amounts of fiber doesn't guarantee weight loss. Fiber has no absorbable calories, which simply means that high-fiber diets are lower in calories. That's the real reason you lose weight initially on these diets.

However, eating excessive amounts of fiber can be rough on the digestive system. And it may push healthy, nutrient-rich foods out of your system with the fiber, preventing nutrients from being absorbed.

ORNISH PLAN AND PRITIKIN DIET

The Ornish plan limits your protein intake to a mere 15 percent of your total daily calories. It also claims that any calories from fat cause you to get fat. The Pritikin diet forces you to limit fat consumption to less than 10 percent of your total daily calories.

With such low amounts of protein (Ornish plan) or fat (Pritikin diet), it's not likely that you'll feel full on either diet. That's why some people overeat on these plans or can't stick to the program for any great length of time.

POINT PLANS AND PREPARED MEALS

Some weight loss plans limit the amount you eat by assigning you points based on your body weight and weight loss goals. The challenge with that is if you're not careful, you can gobble up all your points in one or two meals. That may leave you starving later in the day.

There are also diet plans that require you to buy packaged meals. On these plan, dieters often find themselves at a loss for what to eat when they aren't at home because they're not taught how to create their own healthy meals. Plus these plans can be pricey. Chances are, it's your bank account that will decide when you quit.

CHAPTER 3

Low-Carb Diets Don't Work

I believe that low-carbohydrate, high-protein diets, such as the Atkins diet, the South Beach Diet, and the Zone Diet, are as unhealthy and dangerous as any fad diet. But because they have been immensely popular for the past decade, I feel they deserve a chapter of their own.

So what is a high-protein, low-carb diet? It's any diet that stresses eating lots of protein (such as meat and eggs) while severely limiting carbohydrates (such as bread, potatoes, pasta, and rice). Most low-carb diets also make you avoid fruits, vegetables, and other good-for-you foods.

WHAT YOU LOSE—BESIDES WEIGHT—ON THESE DIETS

What's made low-carb diets so popular is that you do drop off pounds— at least in the short term. But instead of losing fat, these are the five things you're losing on a low-carb diet.

1. WATER
Although low-carb, high-protein diets cause a sudden weight loss initially, much of what you're losing is water. When you starve yourself of carbs, your body is left with no choice but to use up its glycogen, which is the stored carbohydrates it keeps on reserve to fuel activity. Each gram of glycogen has 3 to 4 grams of water attached to it, so as your body uses it up, excess water is shed, and the needle on the scale starts to move downward. The problem is, as soon as you go back to eating normally, your body restocks glycogen—and the excess water—so the weight comes right back.

2. MUSCLE
After its initial water-weight loss, your body has to turn elsewhere to find calories to fuel activity. That's when it starts gobbling up any lean muscle and organ tissue it can find as a source of energy.

3. NUTRIENTS AND FIBER
Most low-carb diets limit the amount of fresh fruits and vegetables you can eat. This leaves your body severely deficient in vitamins and minerals, not to mention dietary fiber.

4. INTEREST
Because so many foods (fruits, cereals, breads, grains, starches, baked goods, dairy products, starchy vegetables, and sweets) are eliminated or severely limited, this kind of diet is very hard to incorporate into life on a long-term basis. After a few weeks of following any low-carb regime, you'll lose interest in the diet because you're constantly feeling hungry and unsatisfied with the food you're allowed to eat.

5. YOUR HEALTH
Some low-carb diets let you eat large amounts of foods that are extremely high in saturated fats. That's why the American Heart Association warns that low-carb diets can raise your cholesterol levels and increase your risk of heart disease, stroke, and diabetes. Recent research suggests that low-carb diets may contribute to certain kinds of cancer.

A low-carb diet can also put an enormous strain on your kidneys. Without carbohydrates to use for fuel, your body switches into a metabolic state called ketosis. When you're in ketosis, you get your energy from ketones—a form of carbon that's created from the breakdown of fat. That sounds like exactly what you're looking for, right? Wrong! It's dangerous to your health. The more ketones you have in your system, the harder your kidneys have to work to filter them, and that can lead to kidney failure. If you already have kidney problems, the situation can be dire: A Harvard study published in the *Annals of Internal Medicine* found that low-carb diets can cause a permanent loss of kidney function in people with reduced kidney function.

WHY LOW-CARB DIETS WON'T WORK LONG TERM

Most people don't experience the negative long-term consequences of low-carb diets only because they quit the diets after just a few weeks. I'd hate to see you waste your time, so take a look at the top five reasons people stop following low-carb diets.

1. THEY'RE FAR TOO COMPLEX

How did you fare in algebra back in high school? Adhering to a low-carb diet requires understanding your body's metabolism and calorie break-downs, choosing the right portion sizes, and dividing up how many grams of protein, carbs, and fats are in every single food you eat. Some of the recipes in these diet books are so complex, they require more cooking skills—and time—than the average person has.

The 5-Factor Diet Difference: With the 5-Factor Diet, the recipes are as tasty as those you'd find in the trendiest Hollywood restaurants, but they're still designed so that anyone—no matter how limited his or her culinary skills—can whip up nutritious meals and snacks with little effort. And as for math, you can count to 5, can't you? Because that's all I'll ever ask you to do.

2. THEY TAKE UP TOO MUCH TIME

Because of their complexity, low-carb diets simply require too much time to think, organize, and implement. That's why many people give up on low-carb diets early on.

The 5-Factor Diet Difference: My clients' time is extremely limited and incredibly valuable. So is yours. I realize that the only way to keep you eating right is to make it easier to eat right. That's why all of the recipes in the 5-Factor Diet take no more than 5 minutes of prep time before cooking.

3. THEY AREN'T VERY SOCIAL

Eating a meal should be a social experience, yet low-carb diets leave many people feeling like the odd man out. You can't enjoy a meal at a restaurant with your friends when you're too busy trying to find a low-carb option on the menu and calculating protein grams. That's why most people end up cheating on these diets when they go out to eat.

The 5-Factor Diet Difference: Most of my celebrity clients work in an industry that practically forces them to be sociable. At the same time, however, privacy is very important to them. Like you, they need a diet program they can use anywhere *without* advertising the fact that they're dieting. The 5-Factor Diet works at home, on the road, or in any restaurant, so you'll never again have to choose between food and friends.

4. THEY DON'T SHOW YOU HOW TO EXERCISE

Low-carb diets may mention how essential exercise is for losing weight, but none of them go into detail about how you should exercise. That's like telling people a road trip will be much faster and smoother if they buy a faster engine, and then never saying where to find one!

The 5-Factor Diet Difference: The 5-Factor Diet is one of the few nutritional programs out there that show you the right way to eat *and* the right way to exercise.

5. THEY SLOW YOU DOWN ON EVERY LEVEL

Your brain relies on carbohydrates to help it function. Yet these low-carb diets reduce the amount of carbs you eat to a trickle of what your brain desperately needs. No wonder low-carb, high-protein dieters tend to have a tough time concentrating. They also end up suffering from fatigue, which leaves them with less energy for exercise.

The 5-Factor Diet Difference: With the 5-Factor Diet, not only will you be free to eat carbohydrates, but you'll also learn which ones are best for your body. And while other diets may shock you when you see what you *can't* eat, with my 5-Factor Diet, you'll be amazed at what you *can* eat.

BEWARE OF THESE POPULAR LOW-CARB DIETS

You've just heard all the negatives that low-carb diets have in common, but each version is also controversial for a variety of its own reasons. Here are the facts you deserve to know.

ATKINS DIET

This popular low-carb diet contends that overconsumption of carbohydrates is the main reason for obesity. Bread, pastas, and potatoes are to be avoided on this plan. Therefore, the Atkins diet severely restricts how many carbohydrates you eat each day and limits your daily calories to between 1,200 and 1,800. The reason this diet is appealing to many people is that you do lose a certain amount of weight—plus you can eat fatty meats, certain fried foods, high-fat dairy products, cheese, eggs, and even butter.

All the freedom the Atkins diet offers comes at a price. Because it's so anti-carb, the diet is lacking in fruits, whole grains, and fiber. Your body misses out on many important nutrients, including vitamin B, vitamin C, and other phytonutrients that boost your immune system. You may drop a few quick pounds by stripping most carbohydrates from your diet, but it's mostly water weight and muscle tissue—and it may place you at risk for a series of short- and long-term health problems.

Your risk of developing osteoporosis may increase because the diet lowers your calcium intake. Research published in the *American Journal of Kidney Disease* found that healthy subjects who tried the Atkins diet experienced calcium losses that were 65 percent greater than normal.

Your risk of heart disease may increase because the diet encourages people to eat fatty meats and certain cheeses, which are high in artery-blocking saturated fats.

Further, according to the National Weight Control Registry, which monitors the diets of more than 2,500 people who have maintained a 30-pound weight loss for at least a year, fewer than 1 percent of these successful dieters use a low-carb, high-protein plan that resembles the Atkins diet.

ZONE DIET

The Zone Diet is a rigid high-protein, low-carb diet. It requires you to divide every single meal you eat using a 40/30/30 ratio: 40 percent carbohydrate, 30 percent protein, and 30 percent fat.

According to the Zone's creator, most people suffer from insulin imbalances that cause them to put on weight. By eating protein, carbs, and fats in the right proportions, you can correct this imbalance and drop the pounds, along with your risk of developing cardiac diseases, diabetes, depression, cancer, and even PMS.

In order to benefit from the diet, you must follow the calculations to the absolute letter. Dividing the components of every meal you eat can be incredibly complicated and takes the enjoyment out of eating, unless you find pleasure in having to pass a math exam each time you want a meal. This plan is too difficult for anyone with a life to manage, or just to put up with for very long.

I'm sure you have friends who swear by the Zone. I will admit that I've seen people get excited when they lose some weight at the start of the plan. But it's the reduction of total daily calories—1,000 to 1,700 calories a day—that's responsible for the weight loss, not the whole 40/30/30 breakdown. A good portion of the weight loss is water and muscle tissue—two things your body can't afford to lose.

The portion sizes of the carbohydrates you're allowed to eat are so small, you'll forget you even ate them in the first place. Your body won't remember the carbs either, and as a result, you'll never achieve satiety. When you quit this diet you'll have better division skills, but don't count on having a leaner, healthier body.

SOUTH BEACH DIET

The South Beach Diet claims to be different from the Atkins diet because it's not completely anti-carbs; instead it encourages you to eat the "right" kinds of carbs.

The first stage of this three-stage diet requires you to stop eating potatoes, pasta, bread, candy, cookies, alcohol, ice cream, baked goods, and sugar. But giving up all of these vices at once is nearly impossible. It's ironic that the South Beach Diet starts off by saying how the Zone Diet is not the answer and the Atkins diet is too severe. Yet once you look at it carefully, you'll realize South Beach is a mix of Atkins and Zone. And the third and final stage is just the daily allowances recommended by the American Dietetic Association.

South Beach also claims that you'll drop 8–13 pounds in its first two-week phase. But just like on the Atkins diet, you're losing water and not fat.

CHAPTER 4

The 5-Factor Diet Does Work

Take a deep breath and relax. I want you to know that you're finally about to embark on a diet plan that—unlike the fad diets I've shown you don't work in the long term—you can use for the rest of your life. The only side effect of the 5-Factor Diet is a healthier, fitter body. The only danger is that you may stop traffic when you walk downtown. If you're ready for those kinds of results, let's get started.

Many celebrity trainers handle only the exercise portion of their clients' fitness programs. I incorporate both exercise and nutritional information. In fact, that's the core of my business as I work with thousands of people face-to-face, over the phone, and online. I work with people who live all over the world, from South America and Europe to North America, Asia, and Australia. That global perspective has shown me that people eat badly all over the world. I had to create a diet plan that would address the fitness and nutritional needs of anyone, no matter where he or she is from or what his or her nutrition habits and culture.

THE 5-FACTOR DIET IS BASED ON WELL-ESTABLISHED SCIENCE

Most fad diets will base their entire eating plan on one study; other diets take one specific scientific finding and spin an entire eating plan around it. That's not very balanced, is it? Those kinds of programs can never deliver the realistic, healthy diet you need.

The 5-Factor Diet is different. Its components are based on well-established science and on many sound, time-honored studies. These aren't studies that will be refuted six months after this book is published. The 5-Factor Diet and 5-Factor Recipes are supported by unchallenged and rock-solid research that has existed for years—in some cases, the studies were done long before I worked with my first client. (See "5-Factor Golden Rules," page 41, for more on the science behind this diet.) And the 5-Factor Diet is easy to follow: Anyone can use it and see results—no matter who you are or where you're from.

YOU'LL LEARN TO LOVE THE NUMBER 5

The 5-Factor Diet starts and ends with the number 5. In fact, everything in the 5-Factor Diet revolves around the number 5. Here's how my menu plan breaks down—in 5s, of course—to help you stay on track.

5 IS THE NUMBER OF MEALS YOU'LL EAT EVERY DAY

There is no skipping meals on the 5-Factor Diet—and with recipes as tasty as the ones I have developed for you, you won't want to pass up a single bite. Each day, you'll eat your typical three meals (breakfast, lunch, and dinner) plus two healthy snacks, one in midmorning and one in midafternoon.

To figure out when you should eat, start by adding up how many hours you're awake during the day—from the time you get out of bed until you turn out the light at night—and divide that number by 5. The resulting number is roughly the number of hours I want you to wait between meals. For example, if you get up at 7 a.m. and go to bed at 11 p.m., you're awake for 16 hours. Divide 16 by 5 and you get a little over three hours, so you should eat at 8 a.m., 11 a.m., 2 p.m., 5 p.m., and 8 p.m.

As you can already imagine, eating 5 meals a day ensures that you'll never feel hungry or deprived. (In "5 Meals a Day Are Key," page 35, I'll get into more detail about the science behind why eating 5 meals is vital to seeing the best results.)

5 IS HOW MANY ELEMENTS EACH MEAL SHOULD INCLUDE
That may sound daunting, but it's easier than it sounds. There are no particular foods I want you to eat. Rather, I want you to make sure every meal or snack you eat is a mix of five elements: protein, low- to moderate-glycemic carbohydrates, healthy fats, and fiber, along with a sugar-free beverage to wash it down. This is the heart of the 5-Factor Diet.

I'll go into more detail soon, but for now just know that *you* get to decide what foods to eat from these five categories. All I ask is that you incorporate all five on your plate at every meal. To make it effortless, the recipes in this book (see "5-Factor Recipes," page 110) all meet the 5-Factor criteria. If you follow my menu, it'll be easy to stick to the 5-Factor Diet.

5 IS THE MAXIMUM NUMBER OF STEPS, MINUTES, AND MAIN INGREDIENTS EACH RECIPE REQUIRES
I know one of the hardest things about dieting is learning how to prepare what's healthy. With my 5-Factor Diet, I've removed that problem from the equation. Every one of my recipes uses 5 or fewer core ingredients, requires 5 steps or fewer to prepare, and takes only 5 minutes to prepare (not counting cook time). Now you'll always have time to watch what you eat.

Ben Foster   ACTOR, STAR IN THE MOVIE *X-MEN: THE LAST STAND*

"Harley Pasternak has developed an extraordinary program for health and fitness. No trends, no gimmicks. Only serious results. It's user friendly, and it is the most effective way to ensure long-term health."

5 IS HOW MANY DAYS A WEEK YOU SHOULD EXERCISE

Exercise is the important factor that most diets gloss over, yet it's critical in the battle to lose weight and make your body healthy, strong, and more injury resistant. I said this in my first book, *5-Factor Fitness*: Eating is 50 percent of the getting-fit equation, and exercise is the other 50 percent.

To get the full benefit of the 5-Factor Diet, you must exercise. That's why I've included a "New 5-Factor Hollywood Workout" (see page 82) with the 5-Factor Diet. It makes it easy to exercise five days a week, so you will always feel great while maximizing your progress.

5 IS THE NUMBER OF FOOD TYPES YOU'LL STOCK IN YOUR KITCHEN

As part of the 5-Factor Diet, I have determined the 5 types of foods— proteins, carbohydrates, condiments, snacks, and beverages—that you should always have on hand. I've further broken this down into the 5-Factor Must-Have Foods, comprising are five of the best nutritional picks from each category, for 25 essential foods you'll always want to have on hand. (For details, see "5-Factor Must-Have Foods," page 50.) There's no guesswork with my eating plan.

WHY THE 5-FACTOR DIET WILL WORK FOR YOU

I call my plan the 5-Factor Diet, but truth be told, it's not as much a diet as a lifestyle. It works for a number of reasons, all of which should resonate with you, especially if you've ever failed at dieting in the past. It works because I can make the following five important promises to you.

1. YOU'LL NEVER FEEL HUNGRY OR DEPRIVED

Have you ever been on a diet that gives you a feeling of emptiness in your stomach, as if you haven't eaten for weeks? That sensation simply doesn't exist on my 5-Factor Diet for several reasons. One of the main principles behind the 5-Factor Diet is eating 5 times a day. It's hard to be hungry with 5 meals a day!

Eating 5 meals spaced evenly throughout the day also keeps your blood sugar (also called blood glucose) stable, which naturally keeps your appetite in check. I've found that eating frequent meals has an impor- tant effect on eating habits. My clients tell me that they always feel as if they're either just about to eat, eating, or just finishing a meal. That's good because it means they never feel desperate for food.

Another reason you won't feel hungry is that you'll combine five very important things—protein, low- or moderate-glycemic carbs, fiber, healthy fats, and a sugar-free beverage—in every meal. (See "The Ideal 5-Factor Meal," page 42, for more details.) These five foods work with one another not just to improve your health and help you lose weight but also to leave you feeling fuller.

Never feeling hungry or deprived is exactly the condition I want for you, because that will keep you from eating more than you should. In studies, critical hospital patients who were given the option to administer their own morphine for pain actually chose to use less than what their doctors would have given them. Similarly, you may find you eat less on the 5-Factor Diet simply because it puts *you* in control— instead of dictating exactly what you can and can't have.

> **MY 5-FACTOR DIET PROMISES**
>
> 1. You'll never feel hungry or deprived.
> 2. You'll enjoy a "cheat" day every week.
> 3. You don't have to buy supplements.
> 4. You won't spend hours in the kitchen.
> 5. You can use the 5-Factor Diet everywhere you go.

The 5-Factor Diet isn't based on restrictions. You won't be cutting carbs or eliminating sugar or any entire food group. In fact, half of this book is filled with recipes for delicious pizza, spaghetti, pancakes, burritos, and many other dishes that most people crave. And it's easy to fit the foods you like into the 5-Factor Diet even if you don't follow my recipes all the time.

2. YOU'LL ENJOY A "CHEAT" DAY EVERY SINGLE WEEK

On the 5-Factor Diet, you're rewarded each week with the chance to eat whatever you want—guilt free. Why would any diet allow you to do such a thing?

You must remember this: Living healthfully should not come at the expense of living well. I think it's awfully sad when somebody refuses to eat her own birthday cake. Or when someone visits the most delicious French restaurant in New York City but orders only a green salad because he's dieting. I would ask those people, "Why are you alive? What good is your health if you aren't enjoying life?" The 5-Factor program never forgets that.

Common GRAMMY NOMINATED MUSICIAN, ACTOR

"Being trained by Harley has made me realize that physical fitness is part of the spirit, body, and mind connection. His insight and energy toward training and health have been a blessing toward improving my life."

Everyone needs a mini meal vacation, if you will. Taking off one day a week is a catharsis. It's a mental relief. It re-empowers you, so you never feel like you're in a diet prison. In fact, an occasional high-calorie day may be just what your body needs to lose weight. Researchers at the National Institutes of Health discovered that subjects who for one day ate twice as many calories as they do normally increased their metabolism by 9 percent in the 24 hours that followed. So cheating one day can help you burn calories—as long as you return to the plan the next day.

If you're worried that cheating may make you want to stray the next day as well, don't fret. Most likely, the cheat day is exactly what you need to prove how well the 5-Factor Diet is working.

It's a lot like using premium fuel in your car. You don't realize how well your car runs on it until the day you decide to save a dime and pour in a few gallons of cheap fuel instead. Suddenly your car sputters and the motor doesn't seem to respond as well. It'll be the same for you when you put away the premium 5-Factor Recipes and fill up on junk.

That's one of the advantages to a cheat day. I want you to cheat so you can see how sluggish you feel when you slip back into old habits. I guarantee that after a few cheats, you'll begin to ask yourself afterward, "Was that really worth it?" You may find yourself craving pizza all week and then, after you have it, realize the main reason you craved it was because you weren't allowed to have it. I can tell you that after my cheat day, I feel mentally and physically different in a way that reminds me how much healthier my body feels when I follow the 5-Factor Diet.

You can pick any one day of the week to splurge, but I suggest you try to make it the same day each week so you always have something to look forward to. Of course, if you know there's a day in the week that's going to be more of a challenge foodwise—perhaps you've been invited to a party or you have a work dinner—then feel free to switch days.

Personally, I prefer Sunday for my cheat day because it's usually a day that's more social, and a day when I'm more likely to be around the sinful foods I've been dodging diligently all week. For me, Sunday also feels like the official end of the week. By making their cheat day Sunday, many of my clients feel as if they are building up to something that they earn through sticking to the plan.

3. YOU DON'T NEED SUPPLEMENTS

It strikes me as odd that so many people are willing to shell out large amounts of money for flavorless pill and powder supplements to add nutrients to their diets—nutrients they could be getting simply by eating the right combination of foods. Those foods would also fill them up so they wouldn't binge on the nutritionless fare that was causing them to be nutrient deprived in the first place.

While writing this book, I looked up the word *supplement* in the dictionary. By definition, it's "something added to make up for a deficiency." If you're eating the right foods according to the 5-Factor Diet, you never have to worry about being deficient in any nutritional area, and you never have to spend a dime on supplements. The 5-Factor Diet is based on the inherent nutritional value of real foods. It is designed to give you the right amount of macro- and micronutrients that your body needs—nutrients you may not be getting from your diet right now. (If you have an allergy or a religious obligation that prevents you from eating a particular food—such as eggs, milk, or shellfish—the 5-Factor Diet offers plenty of other options that are equally abundant in nutrients. That way, you can tailor the diet to accommodate your needs without missing out on nutrition.)

Is it OK to take a multivitamin while on the 5-Factor Diet? Of course it is. In fact, I encourage you to take multivitamins, but not because the 5-Factor Diet is deficient. Certain foods—especially fruits, vegetables, and

> **"I'm a baseball player with the Los Angeles Dodgers, and the 5-Factor program has changed my life. I ended up losing 40 pounds before spring training, and the level of fitness that I have achieved has helped me have the best season of my career. 5-Factor has become my off-season and in-season training program. Thanks, Harley!"**
>
> **Casey Hoorelbeke** WEIGHT LOST SO FAR: **40 lbs.**

meats—can lose a percentage of their vitamins and minerals, depending on how they're prepared or when they're picked. A multivitamin serves as backup insurance for your body, just in case some of your foods have reduced levels of micro- and macronutrients.

Most people can choose a regular over-the-counter multivitamin from the drugstore. However, women who are no longer menstruating, as well as men, should choose types that don't contain iron.

There are a few supplements that can make life easier because of their convenience. For example, if you simply can't get your hands on another protein source to include in a meal, I encourage you to use protein powders and high-protein RTD (Ready to Drink) meal replacement drinks. In fact, I put RTDs on my list of "5-Factor Must-Have Foods" (page 61).

4. YOU WON'T SPEND HOURS IN THE KITCHEN

Who has time to bake a casserole? I don't, my clients don't, and I'm sure you don't either. Whether you're the head of a corporation or the head of your household, time is tight for everyone. Lack of time is a big reason why a lot of us eat badly to begin with. It often seems far easier and faster to swing by a drive-through or grab a packaged snack than it is to prepare a healthy dish from scratch.

It's a myth that cooking healthy has to take lots of time. To prove that fact, I designed all the 5-Factor Recipes in this book to be prepared in five minutes or less. How is that possible? Every recipe has a maximum of 5 key ingredients. Each recipe has 5 or fewer steps to follow. With the 5-Factor Diet, you can stop watching the clock and start watching your shrinking waistline.

Even if you decide to create your own tasty dishes in addition to mine, you'll see how every food I've recommended for you to eat is easy to prepare. And because you don't count calories or portion sizes with the 5-Factor Diet, you don't waste time worrying about anything but enjoying your food.

5. YOU CAN USE THE 5-FACTOR DIET EVERYWHERE

Some of my clients are musicians, and when they're on tour they can be in a different city every night. So I needed to create a nutritional plan that they could stick to no matter where they landed the next day. That's perhaps the greatest gift the 5-Factor Diet offers anyone who wants to lose weight: It makes it easy to take your healthy habits with you outside your home and wherever you go.

The 5-Factor Diet doesn't require that you eat certain foods or certain portions. There are no strange supplements to order, no meetings to attend, no refrigerators filled with packaged meals. All you have to do in order to stick to this plan is eat five meals a day, with each meal containing a protein, a low- or moderate-glycemic carbohydrate, fiber, a healthy fat, and a sugar-free beverage.

With so few guidelines, you can see that it's easy to do the 5-Factor Diet anywhere. You can go to Jamaica and have jerk chicken with rice and peas and be eating the 5-Factor Diet. You can head to Spain and have brown rice with seafood. You can take the 5-Factor Diet with you as your own personal travel partner—anywhere in the world—and get results!

5 Meals a Day Are Key

Research has shown that eating five meals a day rather than the traditional three (or two, for those who unwisely skip breakfast) is optimal for maintaining healthy and stable insulin levels.

When I attended the University of Toronto years ago, my professors included Dr. David Jenkins and Dr. Thomas M. S. Wolever. Those names may not mean anything to you—and if they do, then I'm proud of you—but they did to me. You see, Jenkins and Wolever were two of the world's leading active glycemic index (GI) researchers. In fact, it was they who created the glycemic index—the system that measures, on a scale of 0 to 100, the body's blood sugar response to carbohydrates. They also suggested eating smaller meals throughout the day—"grazing" instead of gorging. A few years after that research was published, I was lucky, and honored, to study under both of them. They have had a profound

> "I wanted to lose my belly, but I was completely unmotivated to work out because most programs looked too long and complicated to start. I found 5-Factor to be well structured and extremely easy to maintain. In just eight weeks, I lost approximately 16 pounds and have managed to keep it off!"
>
> Yvon Brunet AGE: **48** WEIGHT LOST SO FAR: **16 lbs.**

influence on me, both personally and professionally. They're the reason you're holding this book.

WHY 5 MEALS A DAY WORKS

It started the day I decided to put my professors' theories to the test. At first I tried eating six meals a day, but I found it didn't feel very natural because I was used to eating breakfast, lunch, and dinner. Trying to squeeze in six meals felt like I was stuffing myself. Five meals is a lot easier and more sensible to maintain. I had my regular breakfast, lunch, and dinner and added snacks in between. As soon as I stuck with 5 meals, I felt—and saw—the results. From there, I researched ways of making my 5 meals even more effective at fighting fat, building muscle, and improving my overall health. The result is the 5-Factor Diet.

By following this 5-meal-a-day plan, you are changing the way you eat and the reasons why you are eating. If you eat on a schedule, rather than waiting until you're hungry and *must* eat, you become proactive with your diet instead of reactive. *You* are in control of what—and how much—you consume. Once you're in that driver's seat, you get to control how your body looks, feels, and performs.

5-FACTOR DIET BENEFITS

When you stick to my 5-meal-a-day 5-Factor Diet, you'll benefit from five important changes to your body that most diets simply can't offer.

1. IT LOWERS YOUR INSULIN LEVELS

Eating 5 meals a day—and eating the right combinations of foods—can prevent your body from releasing excess insulin into its system. By eating 5 normal-size meals instead of the usual two or three big meals, you tend to eat less food at each meal. Eating less food at each meal means you naturally end up eating less sugar. As a result, less insulin is released and you store less fat.

Keeping your insulin levels low all day long isn't important just for losing fat. It's also necessary if you want to avoid the dangerous medical condition hyperinsulinemia, which occurs when you have too much insulin in your blood too often. This condition is harmful to your long-term health. It also affects you daily by lowering your concentration, diminishing your memory, and causing headaches and dizziness. Sticking with the 5-meals-a-day rule of the 5-Factor Diet prevents all of the above problems, so all you have to do is eat instead of worry.

2. IT GIVES YOU MORE ENERGY ALL DAY

Despite all the other health benefits of the 5-Factor Diet, my guess is that your main goal is to lose weight. Following my system certainly will make that happen. But what really gives you an edge over other dieters is the enormous amount of energy you'll have on this plan. Eating 5 smaller meals a day keeps a nice, steady stream of calories flowing, so you feel more energized and less sluggish. Eating larger meals less often has the exact opposite effect—Thanksgiving, anyone?

You also get an energy boost on the 5-Factor Diet because you're eating protein at all 5 meals. Here's why: One of protein's most important amino acids is tyrosine, which can increase your mental alertness and energy by elevating the brain chemicals dopamine and norepinephrine. By eating protein 5 times a day as opposed to two or three times a day, you release these chemicals twice as often for extra energy all day. That's a nutritional secret many fad dieters—and even the general population, for the most part—never take advantage of. How many times have you seen someone snack on pretzels, fruits, or other carbohydrates without eating anything else with it? When it comes to staying energized, that's a big no-no.

What you decide to do with your newfound energy is up to you. Maybe you'll use it to exercise more effectively. Or maybe you'll use that extra burst to get more done at work or focus on a relationship. Whatever you do, I promise you'll have energy when you need it—always.

3. IT IGNITES YOUR METABOLISM

Did you know that you burn more calories eating than when you're at rest? It's ironic but true. Every time you eat, your body uses up a certain amount of energy—and calories—digesting, absorbing, metabolizing, and storing your meal. In fact, about 5 to 15 percent of your total calories is spent on digestion alone. It's called the "thermic effect of food" (TEF): The more often you eat, the more often your metabolism revs up as your body processes the food. That's yet another scientific reason why there are five meals spaced throughout the day in the 5-Factor Diet.

I like to think of the metabolism as a pinwheel—you know, the toy that looks like a mini fan on a stick that spins when you blow air through it. Your metabolism is like a pinwheel, and you want to keep it spinning. The faster and longer you can make it spin, the more calories you burn.

Each time you eat a meal, it's like blowing air on a pinwheel. If you wait too long before blowing again, the pinwheel starts to slow down. To keep your metabolism constantly spinning, you must time your meals so that just as your body begins to slow down, more food arrives to revive it. Eating 5 meals a day keeps these breezes flowing and your metabolism spinning.

> **5-FACTOR DIET BENEFITS**
>
> 1. It lowers your insulin levels.
> 2. It gives you more energy all day.
> 3. It ignites your metabolism.
> 4. It improves your mood.
> 5. It reduces stress.

My diet gives you even more of a TEF advantage because of the foods you eat at each meal. Protein has a TEF roughly twice as high as that of carbohydrates and fat. That's why simply raising the amount of protein you eat daily from 15 percent of your total calories (the amount most people eat) to 35 percent (the amount I want you to eat) will increase your TEF by 21 calories daily. That number may seem tiny, but remember, the effect is cumulative.

4. IT IMPROVES YOUR MOOD

Have you ever felt agitated, depressed, or irritable during the day, but you couldn't pinpoint what was causing it? It might be from eating less often than you should—something eating 5 meals a day can fix.

John Mayer <small>GRAMMY-WINNING SINGER AND SONGWRITER</small>

"5-Factor is not a diet, in the sense that there's nothing to fall off of. There's nothing to say good-bye to, and nothing to long for. It is almost too good to be true!"

I've explained that eating less often and having bigger meals raises your insulin levels so you end up storing excess calories as fat. There's also an emotional downside to this situation. When you eat less often and have larger meals, your body not only releases insulin but also overcompensates by releasing too much insulin, just to be sure it's doing its job. The result is that your body removes more blood sugar than necessary, causing a net deficit in your body's supply of glucose. Having less energy leaves you feeling less happy and more miserable, no matter how happy you normally are. Eating 5 smaller meals a day can prevent this and improve your mood—unless you have a good reason to be angry or upset!

On the 5-Factor Diet, you're also protecting yourself from mood swings by eating a low- to moderate-glycemic carbohydrate at every meal. Research performed at the Massachusetts Institute of Technology found that eating less than 50 grams of carbohydrates daily can cause a significant drop in the chemical serotonin, which your brain releases to help regulate mood and appetite.

When your serotonin level dips, you're more susceptible to feeling depressed and anxious. Getting enough serotonin on a regular basis raises how much of the chemical your body produces. Eating 5 meals a day—with carbs at each meal—keeps your levels steady so you never encounter the kind of emotional highs and lows you may have felt on other diets.

The 5-Factor Diet and 5-Factor Recipes also incorporate plenty of foods that are rich in folate—a mineral that helps lower homocysteine, an amino acid that's been shown to cause depression at high levels—as well as healthy fats and essential fatty acids, which have been shown to help naturally treat depression.

5. IT REDUCES STRESS

Eating is important for a reason most people don't quite understand: It's a time to relax and put your life on pause for a moment. A meal is a time for reflection for many people—or at least it should be. It's a time to rest and think.

I want you to look at each meal as "your" time. No matter how stressful your day is, or how angry your boss is making you, I want you to use your five mealtimes to simply pause and ponder, even if it's only for a few minutes. Taking a break isn't just healthy for your mind; it's also beneficial to your body. Taking the time to make a meal, then sit down and eat it, forces you to do something that you might not do otherwise during the day.

As a workaholic, I made a New Year's resolution a few years ago to find a balance in life. I wanted to speak to my parents more often. I wanted to read more. I wanted to spend more time focusing on me instead of all the work that was always piling up around me.

I used my 5 meals a day as a no-excuse way to live up to that promise. They gave me five opportunities in the day to reach out and say hello to my mother or read a chapter in a book. They helped bring balance to my day. I felt calmer and less stressed by the time each meal was over.

Studies have shown that the more stressful your life is, the higher your odds of being overweight. A study performed at the New York Academy of Sciences found that most women who face chronic stress suffer from a condition called stress overeating, caused by the hormone cortisol, which your body releases when under stress. Not only is cortisol toxic to your immune system, but it stimulates appetite, which may be why the study's subjects overate during stressful times.

A study from Yale University found that women dealing with stress typically may develop excess fat around their waistlines and surrounding their organs. The study theorized that there are more cortisol-sensitive receptors within fat cells in your belly than any other areas of your body. That means stressing out about your belly could keep you from losing it—if you don't find the time to unwind, that is.

Exercising regularly and adhering to a healthy diet can lower your stress and help keep your cortisol levels low. Of course, those are both things you'll be doing naturally when you follow my 5-Factor Diet. Taking the time to reflect with each meal can help curb your daily stress even further, helping you keep off the fat.

CHAPTER 6

5-Factor Golden Rules

When I was a graduate student doing nutrition research for Canada's Department of National Defense, I learned all about the biochemistry of food and its effects on the body. What always amazed me was that amid all the science, there were 5 clear-as-day factors that were universally ideal for losing weight, maintaining lean muscle, and improving overall health. It is these 5 rules that became the scientific basis for my 5-Factor Diet.

THE SCIENCE BEHIND THE 5-FACTOR DIET

Scientific factor #1. Protein is the building block of the most important parts of our bodies, from muscles, hormones, and enzymes to skin, organs, and blood.

Scientific factor #2. All carbohydrates are not created equal, as proven by the glycemic index, which is the system that measures on a scale of 0 to 100 the body's blood sugar response to carbohydrates. It's healthier to avoid foods ranked high on the glycemic index and eat low-glycemic carbohydrates instead.

Scientific factor #3. Fiber is vital to the body, as proven by overwhelming research: It has the power to lower everything from bad cholesterol and blood pressure to the risk of certain types of cancers. It also helps keep your digestive system regular.

Scientific factor #4. Not all fats are evil. In fact, healthy fats are an important part of a good diet. Studies show that our hormones, nerves, reproductive system, skin, and hundreds of other parts of the body rely on fat to function properly—yet our society desperately tries to remove every last bit of fat from our foods.

Scientific fact #5. Water is essential to life. Unfortunately, many people use thirst as an excuse to consume sugar and excessive calories.

Using these scientific and nutritional facts, I created the 5-Factor Diet, which—unlike fad diets—is guaranteed to stand the test of time.

THE IDEAL 5-FACTOR MEAL

My diet works because it combines the right 5 types of foods—protein, carbohydrates, fiber, healthy fats, and beverages—in each meal. Each of these 5 Factors is critical to your nutritional success. It's simple: At every meal eat one food from each of the five categories. It's a program that's nutritionally sound and easy to use for the rest of your life.

> **5-FACTOR FOODS FOR EVERY MEAL**
> 1. Protein
> 2. Low- to moderate-GI carbohydrates
> 3. Fiber
> 4. Healthy fats
> 5. Sugar-free beverages

Think of every 5-Factor Diet meal as a shopping trip to a five-story department store, which you can't leave until you've purchased something from all five floors. That's the simplicity of the 5-Factor Diet, only instead of a store, it's your plate. Instead of having to buy something from every floor, you must eat something from the five 5-Factor food categories.

It's the easiest and simplest way to move toward a leaner, healthier body. Here is a closer look at each food category, with all the details on why it's important and information on proper portion size.

1. PROTEIN

Every meal or snack should contain a low-fat protein such as chicken breast, fish, seafood, egg whites, or cottage cheese. Aim for one-third of your total calories to come from protein, which is vital for maintaining muscle tissue and regulating metabolism.

Protein is No. 1 on this list for several good reasons. First, it helps you feel fuller longer. In recent studies, subjects who ate high-protein, moderate-carbohydrate meals (which is exactly what's recommended in the 5-Factor Diet and the breakdown of every 5-Factor Recipe you'll find in this book) had a greater feeling of fullness after meals that lasted longer during the day than did subjects who ate high-fat meals. That's because there's a certain amount of fat found in animal-based protein like chicken or fish. That may sound like a step in the wrong direction if you want to lose fat, but staying fuller for a longer period of time can curb your hunger in between meals.

EAT THE 5-FACTOR DIET ANYWHERE!

You don't have to stray from the 5-Factor Diet when dining out. Here are a few of my favorite combinations to order at different-style restaurants.

IF YOU'RE DINING ...	ORDER ...
American	Turkey burger
Canadian	Grilled ostrich and a bowl of lentil soup
Chinese	Black bean and shrimp stir-fry
Cuban	Fish soup or grilled chicken with black beans
Greek	Chicken shish kabob or Greek salad
Indian	Tandoori chicken with basmati rice
Italian	Branzino, minestrone soup, or tomato-basil salad
Jamaican	Jerk chicken breasts or rice and beans
Japanese	Seaweed salad, miso soup, sashimi, or teriyaki chicken
Mexican	Chicken fajitas

Because protein helps you maintain muscle, it also helps raise your resting metabolism. It takes more calories to maintain muscle than fat, so the more muscle you have, the more calories you burn throughout the day. Eating plenty of protein and following the 5-Factor Hollywood Workout will help you build more muscle, thus revving up your metabolism.

The best perk about protein is that out of the three macronutrients—protein, carbohydrates, and fat—it's the most difficult to store as body fat. When you eat more fat than your body needs, your body stores it as fat. When you eat more simple carbohydrates than your body needs, blood sugar levels spike. This causes your body to release excess insulin, which helps speed up the conversions of carb calories into fat.

However, when you eat more protein, your body doesn't require as much insulin to metabolize it. Having less insulin in your system lowers your odds of having any excess calories converted to fat. Plus your body has to convert the protein into carbohydrates before it can be converted into fat. All that takes a lot of work, which is why most excess protein leaves the body before it has a chance to become an extra pant size.

The one type of protein I don't recommend is nuts. Some nutritionists sing their praises because they are low in carbohydrates, but most nuts, in general, receive greater than three-fourths of their calories from fat. Although nuts are often considered a major protein source, in truth many of them contain only small amounts of low-quality protein that is incomplete (lacking one or more essential amino acids) or is not bio-available (that is, the body can't use it).

Instead of nuts, pick lower-fat, more-complete protein sources such as egg whites, fish, lean beef, chicken breast, turkey breast, and fat-free milk. You'll maximize your intake of quality protein while minimizing your intake of bad fats.

2. CARBOHYDRATES

Every meal should contain a carbohydrate that ranks low or moderate on the glycemic index. Good choices include vegetables, wild rice, beans, lentils, oatmeal, sweet potato, and quinoa.

Carbohydrates have taken a lot of flak lately, thanks to poorly conceived fad diets. The truth is that carbs are responsible for fueling your body and providing most of the energy you need to live. That's why every meal

> **"I had always been interested in fitness, but it wasn't until reading your book that I finally corrected all my mistakes. I was overloading on carbohydrates, eating three meals a day, and didn't know the right balance of protein and carbs. Thanks to 5-Factor, I learned about eating the right types of foods and the benefits of having 5 small meals a day."**
>
> **Michael Bigman** WEIGHT LOST SO FAR: **8 lbs.**

you eat should have at least two portions (that's 50 percent of your total calories) of some type of low- to moderate-glycemic carbohydrate.

Why am I not anti-carb like other nutrition experts? Because eating a mixture of fibrous carbohydrates and protein keeps you sharp. You see, carbohydrates are absorbed into the system much faster than protein is, so eating a mixture of protein and the right carbs increases your alertness by burning calories at staggered times. That gives you a feeling of satiety and an even release of energy throughout the day. That's energy your body can use to exercise later on. Carbs also help the fat in your diet be more efficiently metabolized. Basically, fat burns in a carbohydrate flame. Most low-GI carbohydrates also contain some soluble fiber (see "Fiber," page 46), which is also important.

I've mentioned the glycemic index (GI), which is a system that rates carbohydrate foods based on how quickly your body converts them into glucose. Foods that break down rapidly—such as starchy foods—release glucose quickly into your blood and rank higher on the index. Foods that break down slowly—such as spinach and cabbage—slowly release glucose into your blood, so they rank lower on the index.

The problem with high-glycemic food is that when its sugar enters your blood, your pancreas immediately has to produce insulin to help regulate it. Your body's natural response to extra insulin in your system is to store whatever calories it can find—whether from carbs, protein, or fat—as unwanted body fat.

Low- to moderate-glycemic carbs release glucose at a much slower pace, so your pancreas produces less insulin. Less insulin means less body fat—need I say more? That's what makes low- to moderate-glycemic foods such a critical part of the 5-Factor Diet.

Try to choose carbs with a glycemic level under 80. These foods can give your body enough all-day energy without causing an insulin surge that may store excess body fat. I prefer fruits and vegetables because they're nutrient rich, low in calories, and water based, which means they're packed with water that fills your stomach. Good picks that are low to moderate on the GI scale include apples, black beans, broccoli, cabbage, carrots, celery, cherries, chickpeas, cucumbers, grapefruits, green peas, lentils, lettuce, lima beans, mushrooms, onions, pears, peaches, peppers, plums, oatmeal, oranges, snow peas, spinach, strawberries, sweet potatoes, and wild rice.

3. FIBER
Every meal should contain 5 to 10 grams of fiber. The health benefits of fiber are numerous: It reduces your risk of developing diabetes and some cancers and lowers your overall blood cholesterol. Fiber slows down the release of glucose (again, the substance your body uses for energy) into the bloodstream, preventing your body from burning through its energy stores too quickly. Fiber even increases how quickly your meals pass into your stomach. The faster you can move food through your digestive system, the less fat and calories you'll absorb. But most important, fiber leaves you feeling full, so you end up eating less at every meal.

Fiber comes in two forms: soluble and insoluble. Both are valuable assets, though, for entirely different reasons. Soluble fiber—found in foods such as peas, oat bran, seeds, beans, barley, lentils, and apples—is digestible and helps lower your risk of developing heart disease and high cholesterol. Insoluble fiber—found in wheat bran, whole grains, vegetables, and beans—is not digested or absorbed by your body but passes through instead, which helps improve the health of your digestive system and colon. Insoluble fiber can also help you drop a few extra pounds. A USDA study found that eating 36 grams of fiber each day can prevent your body from absorbing 130 calories a day.

Kanye West SINGER/SONGWRITER

"The 5-Factor Diet saved me on tour. I can't believe there is healthy food that tastes this good. I've never been in better shape!"

You should eat at least 20 to 30 grams of fiber each day. You can have even more than that—if you can handle it—but do make sure you're getting at least the bare minimum by eating 5 grams at each meal. Over your five meals, you'll ensure you're getting at least 25 grams daily. Ideally, I'd like you to eat 10 grams of fiber at breakfast, lunch, and dinner and 5 grams per snack, which would place you right around 40 grams of fiber a day.

That might sound like a lot, but simply throwing a few handfuls of fiber-rich beans (about ½ cup) into a meal adds around 8 grams of fiber. Some of my favorite fiber-rich foods include whole-grain cereal, brown or wild rice, beans and lentils, no-flour wheat breads, and whole veggies and fruits that have edible skins or seeds.

4. HEALTHY FATS

If your meal contains any fat, it should always be a healthy one—either monounsaturated or polyunsaturated. If you believe it's better to avoid eating fats altogether, think again. Your body needs it—even if your No. 1 mission is to lose body fat. Fat is a major source of energy and helps the body absorb vitamins A, D, E, and K. It also provides taste and consistency, and it helps you feel full so you eat less. Research has even shown that having too little fat in the diet can cause clinical depression. That's because to function properly, your brain needs a certain amount of fat, especially the kind containing omega-3 and omega-6 fatty acids.

Besides, I really don't need to remind you to eat fat because it's almost impossible to avoid. But when you're going to eat a food that contains fat or is cooked in fat, you should stick to the healthy kind—or "good fats," as nutritionists like to call them.

GOOD FATS/BAD FATS: SIMPLE SUBSTITUTIONS

Replacing bad fats with good fats doesn't have to be difficult. Here are five ways to do it that your taste buds won't notice but your body will appreciate.

1. Switch your cooking oil to grapeseed, canola, or extra-virgin olive oil. All three work well under extreme heat.

2. Toss a tiny amount of flaxseed meal on your veggies instead of butter or margarine.

3. If a recipe calls for vegetable shortening, substitute half as much virgin olive oil and a dash of salt.

4. Skip packaged snacks like potato chips and eat seeds instead.

5. Instead of using butter or margarine on your food, try extra-virgin olive oil or flaxseed oil mixed with a dash of salt.

Good fats. Monounsaturated fats are good fats because they don't increase your total cholesterol. In fact, they lower your LDL (bad cholesterol) while simultaneously increasing your HDL (good cholesterol). Monounsaturated fats are found in foods such as fish oil, peanut oil, olive oil, and canola oil.

Polyunsaturated fats have the same positive effect, and they're found in a variety of foods, such as fattier fish like mackerel, albacore tuna, rainbow trout, herring, salmon, and sardines, as well as sunflower oil, canola oil, and flaxseed.

Both monounsaturated and polyunsaturated fats may be "healthy," but they are still fat, and eaten in abundance, they will make you fat. To avoid that, limit your fats to 65 grams a day (or 100 grams maximum).

Bad fats. Saturated fats raise your total blood cholesterol and LDL (bad cholesterol). These fats are hard to avoid; if you can't avoid them, eat them sparingly. Saturated fats are found mostly in animal products such as meat, poultry skin, whole milk, butter, milk chocolate, and egg yolks, as well as in coconut oil, palm oil, and palm kernel oil.

Trans fats, or hydrogenated fats, have the same bad effect on your cholesterol. These are synthetic fats created to give a long shelf life to certain foods. You'll find them in processed foods, commercially prepared baked goods, stick butter, margarine, vegetable shortening, and every bad food you've ever seen made with the last two—including french fries and microwave popcorn. I want you to eliminate trans fats from your diet.

5. SUGAR-FREE BEVERAGES

Every meal should be accompanied by a sugar-free beverage such as water, sugar-free soda, tea, coffee, or an unsweetened energy drink. Your goal is to drink 8 to 12 ounces of a healthy beverage with every meal and snack.

Hydration is important for several reasons. First, for every ounce of excess liquid you drink with your meal, that's one ounce of real estate you steal away from food. More liquid in your belly leaves you feeling fuller and lessens your appetite for your next meal—and throughout the day.

Second, you'll burn more calories all day long. Most people are dehydrated and don't even know it. That's because by the time your thirst mechanism kicks in, your body has already lost about 4 to 5 percent of its water. This condition—called chronic mild dehydration—can affect every biochemical function in your body, including digestion. When your body is well hydrated, it can digest your food with less effort, so even less of it gets stored as body fat. Keeping your digestive system running well also helps it absorb more nutrients as it processes your food.

Third, being properly hydrated may prevent you from eating as much during your next meal or snack. Often people eat because they think they're hungry when they are actually thirsty. That's because thirst triggers the same physical responses as hunger. The next time you feel the urge to eat, try satisfying that urge with a sugar-free beverage instead.

Drinking 8 to 12 ounces at each of your 5 meals guarantees that you'll drink between 40 and 60 ounces a day. But it's not enough to only drink at meals. I recommend that you drink a total of 10 to 12 glasses (roughly 96 ounces), spread throughout the day. If drinking straight water doesn't sound enticing, mix in a very small amount of fruit juice for flavor. Also opt for ice-cold water when possible. Ice-cold water forces your body to burn calories to heat the water up to your body temperature. The effect may be slight, but every little bit helps!

CHAPTER 7

5-Factor
Must-Have
Foods

Although my 5-Factor Diet neither prohibits nor advocates any one food or food group, I have scouted out foods that are ideally suited to the 5-Factor Diet. These foods will keep your diet varied, wholesome, and delicious. I call them the 5-Factor Must-Have Foods. If you keep your fridge and pantry stocked with at least a week's worth of these foods, you'll find that following the 5-Factor Diet is easy and convenient.

There are 5 categories of foods you should always have at the ready: proteins, carbohydrates, sugar-free beverages, snacks, and condiments. I've also selected the 5 best choices for each category. These 25 foods are the building blocks for many of the recipes in this book. (See "5-Factor Recipes," page 110.) The beauty of the 5-Factor Must-Have Foods is that you can use your imagination and creativity, combining them to make your own quick and healthy meals that match the 5-Factor Diet formula.

THE 25 ESSENTIAL 5-FACTOR FOODS

Over the years I've figured out what works and what doesn't when it comes to diet. While there are no shortcuts in the pursuit of better nutrition and health, it is possible to keep your palate satisfied and your body in shape—and these 25 foods will help you do just that.

PROTEINS

1. Egg whites. Egg whites are often called the perfect source of protein because your body uses 100 percent of the nutrients they contain. They're also free of saturated fats, excess carbohydrates, and cholesterol, which many high-protein foods are laden with. But the main reason they rank high among my 5-Factor Must-Have Foods is the countless ways you can cook them.

5-FACTOR
MUST-HAVE FOOD
CATEGORIES

1. Proteins

2. Carbohydrates

3. Beverages

4. Snacks

5. Condiments

Egg whites are easier than ever to use when cooking, especially since you no longer have to separate them from the yolk yourself. Many grocery stores sell cartons of already-separated liquid egg whites. They're not only convenient but also pasteurized, so they last longer in the refrigerator and carry less risk of food poisoning.

My top picks: Eggology 100% Egg Whites and Egg Beaters Egg Whites

2. Poultry. I have only two rules when it comes to eating poultry: Choose white meat (which is leaner than dark meat) and remove the skin. Poultry is one of the few foods that you can easily strip fat from, so take full advantage of that perk. And remember that chicken isn't your only choice of poultry. Many people don't think of turkey except around the holidays, but it too is low in fat, high in protein, and loaded with ample amounts of zinc, iron, potassium phosphorus, and B vitamins.

To keep your taste buds interested, buy poultry in a variety of forms: Whole breasts are terrific, but so is ground poultry breast or sliced deli-style poultry (as long as it's all-natural and not heavily processed). Keep in mind that the packaged ground chicken and turkey you see in the grocery store often includes the skin so it can be as high in fat as ground beef. For that reason, it's best to have someone at the meat counter grind a skinless chicken or turkey breast for you.

Eva Mendes ACTRESS AND STAR OF THE MOVIE *HITCH*

"Harley has changed my life. Not only do I feel better than ever, but I now can have guilt-free pizza anytime, and that has made me a happy girl."

My top picks: I don't have a favorite brand, but I recommend that you become friendly with your local butcher. That way, you can specifically ask the butcher for the freshest and best cuts of poultry.

3. Seafood. Seafood should be a staple in every kitchen. Why? It's very low in fat and is packed with protein. Fish also contains healthy omega-3 fatty acids, which research has shown can improve the overall health of your heart, joints, and immune system. Better yet, seafood can have a mood-elevating effect on the brain by boosting levels of dopamine and serotonin, two neurotransmitters that naturally help prevent depression. The only downside of seafood is that some fish, specifically tuna, swordfish, and mackeral, may contain high levels of mercury. It's best to limit your intake of these to twice a week, except for light tuna, which you can have up to three times a week (see below).

My top picks: Salmon, cod, tuna, scallops, shrimp, lobster, squid, and crab. When buying canned tuna, pick the less-expensive versions (chunk light or flaked), which have less than half of the mercury of the more expensive white albacore variety. I love the convenience of StarKist Tuna Creations, which comes in a pouch instead of a can; it's easy to transport and easy to open, there's no water to drain, and it comes preflavored.

4. Dairy. Dairy has unfairly gotten a bad reputation because of its fat content, but it's an excellent source of protein and bone-strengthening calcium. Dairy also helps quell your appetite, according to researchers from the University of California at Davis. They found that study participants who ate meals containing dairy products had a 20 percent increase in an appetite-suppressing hormone called cholecystokinin.

Remember that dairy refers to more than just milk. It also comprises hard and soft cheeses (including cottage cheese and cream cheese), yogurt (plain with no sugar added), and sour cream. Always choose fat-free versions of these foods.

My top picks: Fat-free cheese slices and fat-free yogurt. I also highly recommend Quark, an unripened cheese that's a cross between yogurt and cream cheese. Quark is not only tasty but is a high-protein, low-carb food. It also takes on the flavor of other foods, making it a versatile ingredient in both sweet and savory dishes.

5. Game meats. While I was on a movie set a few years ago, I made a chili dinner for a few of the actors I was training. At the end of the meal, they all raved that it was the most delicious chili they'd ever eaten. It was only then that I revealed that the main ingredient was ground bison. They were stunned that its taste and texture were the same as those of regular beef—and thrilled that the fat content was about half that of beef.

Meats like ostrich, bison, elk, caribou, and venison may sound too exotic to eat, but *game* is actually a relative term. Go to the Far East and some of the more common meats are frog and turtle. Go to Eastern Europe and the Caribbean and it's not unusual to eat ox. So be daring and try game meats, which are often leaner than red meat, very high in protein, and high in iron. Adding them to your diet will make a big difference in your life because they let you enjoy the same tastes and textures as those of traditional beef and fat-laden steaks—without all the nutritional negatives.

Most health food and grocery stores stock game meats in their frozen section. Or look online for dealers that specialize in game meats.

There are two important things to remember when choosing game. One, make sure to read the nutritional label because certain cuts are leaner than others. Two, because game has less fat than regular beef, it's easy to overcook. Shave a few minutes off your usual cook time, or you could turn that bison steak into shoe leather.

My top pick: Intermountain Ostrich Cooperative ostrich burgers

CARBS

1. Beans. Beans are mathematically a perfect food. Not only are they a low-glycemic carbohydrate with a small amount of healthy fats, but they're also high in protein and belly-filling fiber. In fact, one serving of beans (about ½ cup) provides close to 8 grams of fiber, which will leave you feeling more satiated—and less likely to overeat.

With so many varieties to choose from—black, red, kidney, pink, garbanzo, and many more—anyone can find a bean he or she likes. Beans are also perfect as a topping; sprinkle a handful on salads, chili, and soups to add extra fiber and protein to any meal.

My top picks: Most of the brands on the market are good, so pick whatever suits your taste buds. Studies have shown that canned beans have the same nutrient profile as fresh beans, so feel free to choose fresh, dried, frozen, or canned depending on what best fits your lifestyle.

2. Grains. Packed with fiber, grains are terrific because they fill you up and make a great companion to any protein. All forms of grain—including oatmeal, oats, lentils, barley, and brown rice—are good choices. One of my all-time favorites, however, is quinoa (pronounced "keen-wa"). This supergrain isn't a common staple—in fact, it can be difficult to find if your local grocery store doesn't have a large health food section—but it's loaded with about 50 percent more protein than most grains, and it's rich in calcium, iron, and the essential B vitamins.

My top picks: Kashi 7 Whole Grain Pilaf and Quaker Weight Control instant oatmeal

> CARBS
> 1. Beans
> 2. Grains
> 3. Breads
> 4. Vegetables
> 5. Fruit

3. Breads. I know what you're thinking: Bread is heavily processed, low in nutrients, and loaded with bad carbohydrates, so why is this a 5-Factor Must-Have Food? The problem with bread isn't bread itself but the ingredients that it's made from. I recommend that you avoid flour if possible. Luckily, there are several bread products such as tortillas, crackers, and flat bread that are made without flour. These products are made from sprouted grains that are not refined as much as flour. They're easy to spot because most brands will have the term *no-flour* or *flourless* right in the name of the product. These items may be located in the health food section of your supermar-

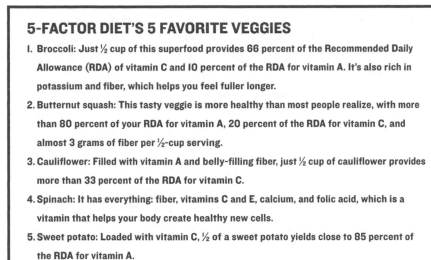

5-FACTOR DIET'S 5 FAVORITE VEGGIES

1. Broccoli: Just ½ cup of this superfood provides 66 percent of the Recommended Daily Allowance (RDA) of vitamin C and 10 percent of the RDA for vitamin A. It's also rich in potassium and fiber, which helps you feel fuller longer.

2. Butternut squash: This tasty veggie is more healthy than most people realize, with more than 80 percent of your RDA for vitamin A, 20 percent of the RDA for vitamin C, and almost 3 grams of fiber per ½-cup serving.

3. Cauliflower: Filled with vitamin A and belly-filling fiber, just ½ cup of cauliflower provides more than 33 percent of the RDA for vitamin C.

4. Spinach: It has everything: fiber, vitamins C and E, calcium, and folic acid, which is a vitamin that helps your body create healthy new cells.

5. Sweet potato: Loaded with vitamin C, ½ of a sweet potato yields close to 85 percent of the RDA for vitamin A.

ket. If your local stores don't carry no-flour breads, a second-best option is to choose breads made with whole grains.

My top picks: Fitness Bread by Mestemacher, Food for Life Ezekiel 4:19 Organic Sprouted Flourless Whole Grain Tortillas, Food for Life Ezekiel 4:19 Sprouted Whole Grain Flourless Cinnamon Raisin Bread

4. Vegetables. Low-calorie, low-glycemic, high in nutrients, and often packed with fiber, vegetables contain disease-fighting antioxidants (vitamins A and C) and potassium, which helps keep your muscles healthy. In short, you simply can't lead a healthy lifestyle if vegetables aren't a regular part of it. You can buy them fresh or frozen and eat them steamed, stir-fried, pureed, or grilled. Just remember that a healthy veggie quickly becomes unhealthy if it's batter-dipped or slathered with high-fat cheese sauce.

Which ones should you eat? Steer clear of avocados, olives, potatoes, and beets, which contain too much fat, carbohydrates, or sugars. All other vegetables are fair game. I prefer to buy mine frozen so I can stock up on all my favorites—and they will keep for months, unlike fresh veggies.

My top picks: Frozen mixed vegetables from Cascadian Farm or Westpac

5. Fruit. USDA research suggests that people who eat more fruit tend to have a lower body mass index (BMI) and lower total body weight than those who eat less fruit. Fruits are fat free and packed with fiber, vitamins, minerals, and antioxidants. Plus they let you enjoy sweet flavors without the empty calories of most sugary foods.

Not all fruits are equal. Some types—such as bananas—are higher on the glycemic index, which means they cause blood sugar levels to surge, thus triggering your body to store body fat. And you don't want that! Don't worry. Here's an easy way to remember which fruits rank low on the glycemic index and are therefore your best choices: The next time you pick up a piece of fruit, ask yourself these three questions. If you answer yes to at least one of them, it's a smart fruit choice:

Does it have edible skin?
(Think of apples, pears, plums, and peaches.)
Does it have edible seeds?
(Think of pomegranates, blackberries, strawberries, and raspberries.)
Is it a citrus fruit?
(Citrus fruits include grapefruit, oranges, and tangerines.)

The only exception to this rule is grapes, which do have an edible skin but are not a good fruit choice due to their high dextrose levels.

My top picks: Fresh fruit is best, but it's smart to keep a backup fruit handy in your freezer. Two of my favorites are Wyman's Quick-Frozen Mixed Fruit and Dole Mixed Berries.

BEVERAGES
1. Water. There's no better beverage than plain, unsweetened water. However, plain, flat water can get boring. To keep things interesting, I tell my clients to buy water in as many different forms as possible. Try sodium-free seltzer and, if you want to spice it up a bit and you're out for a night at a restaurant, sparkling water. Between all the bubbles and the fizz, sparkling water really helps cleanse the palate and adds a different texture.

My top pick: Bottled water and Kellogg's Special K2O Protein Water

2. Coffee. Coffee may sound like an odd choice for my 5-Factor Must-Have Foods, but there's a very important reason I include it. When I was a scientist for the Defense and Civil Institute of Environmental Medicine in Canada, I ran and published scientific studies on the effects of caffeine on exercise. Research has shown that drinking a caffeinated beverage 30 to 90 minutes before exercise can boost your endurance and increase the rate at which your body burns fat. Just keep an eye on how much coffee you drink—I would limit it to no more than three cups a day.

My top pick: Although I don't have a favorite brand, I prefer espresso beverages, such as cappucino and macchiatto. They typically have less than half the caffeine content of regular drip coffee and significantly more taste. The addition of nonfat milk to these beverages adds protein and calcium to your diet. My daily wake-up is usually nonfat espresso macchiatto.

If you do choose to drink regular coffee, keep a close watch on what you put in your cup. Ordinary plain coffee has no calories or sugar, but if you want to sweeten it up, I suggest using fat-free dairy products and Splenda.

3. Tea. Caffeinated tea is another must-have beverage because it offers the same endurance and metabolic benefits as coffee. But tea also comes with its own unique set of health advantages, so stock it in your kitchen, your desk

---

"I had a life-threatening illness and realized that to get through it, I needed to live a much healthier life. Because of its simplicity, 5-Factor allowed me to start while I was in treatment. The 5-Factor plan taught me how doing too much cardio and not eating enough of the right kinds of food combinations make your body hold on to the weight. All of the 5-Factor healthy eating habits helped me beat the illness, and I'm much healthier now."

Trina Jones AGE: **25** WEIGHT LOST SO FAR: **21 lbs.**

---

drawer, and your purse or pocket so you always have a cup when you need it.

Certain teas—especially those that are rich in antioxidants such as polyphenols—have been shown to boost the immune system, ward off colds, soothe aches and pains, and even reduce the risk of developing cancer. One Rutgers University study found that TF-2, a component of black tea, kills colorectal cancer cells without affecting normal healthy cells in the body. The antioxidant polyphenols in some teas can even prevent heart disease. In 2003, USDA researchers found that subjects who drank five cups (there's that magic number again!) of black tea a day for three weeks lowered their LDL (bad) cholesterol by 11 percent.

> **BEVERAGES**
> 1. Water
> 2. Coffee
> 3. Tea
> 4. Sugar-free soda
> 5. Sugar-free juices

As with coffee, drink no more than three cups of caffeinated tea daily. If you drink both coffee and tea, limit your daily consumption of both beverages to three cups total. Once you reach that limit, switch from caffeinated to decaffeinated teas and coffees.

My top picks: Black tea is terrific, but green tea also gets a lot of praise, for good reason. The polyphenols in this centuries-old beverage have been shown to fight certain cancers, ease pain, and burn calories. That's not bad for a few leaves and some water!

Any herbal tea will work fine too. Herbal teas are generally a combination of different herbs—not tea leaves—so they may not offer the same exact health benefits of tea. However, most are still calorie-free, contain different ratios of antioxidants, and offer health benefits that include everything from easing your stomach to relieving depression.

4. Sugar-free sodas. Most people enjoy an ice-cold soda, and that's entirely fine. Not all soda is bad for you. The problem with most sodas is that they are loaded with sugar—some have as much as 42 grams per serving—which can add 100 to 200 unwanted calories to your diet with every can or bottle. Instead, I recommend a no-calorie, Splenda-sweetened soda. That way, you'll stay hydrated and enjoy some flavor with your meal—without throwing on any extra calories. As part of the 5-Factor Diet, though, I would prefer that you limit yourself to one soda a day.

My top picks: Diet 7-Up, Diet Rite, and diet Hansen's Soda, which contains zero caffeine, no sugar, no preservatives, and no artificial flavors or coloring

5. Sugar-free juice. Like most sodas, many juice drinks contain excess sugar despite the fact that their product names sound healthy. That's why I recommend steering clear of any juices that have added sugar. All that sugar means excess calories that your body doesn't need.

My top picks: Fuze drinks, diet Snapple drinks, and diet SoBe drinks

CONDIMENTS

1. Fat-free mayonnaise. Many healthy foods—such as tuna and certain vegetables—can be difficult to swallow because of their blandness. That's why fat-free mayo ranks high on the 5-Factor Must-Have Foods list. It's a "consistency" condiment, adding texture and taste to tuna dishes, chicken salad, salmon salad, and countless other meals.

If you stay away from fat-free mayonnaise because you don't like the taste, then you obviously haven't tried it in a while. Most of the fat-free brands available today actually taste good but without all the cholesterol and high amounts of saturated fat contained in regular mayo.

My top picks: Hellmann's Reduced Fat Mayonnaise and Kraft Fat-Free Mayo

2. Salsa. Just because you're used to eating salsa with bad-for-you foods like nachos doesn't mean this condiment should be banned from your eating routine. A healthy mix of tomatoes, onions, and other vegetables, salsa is all-natural, incredibly low in calories (as low as 4 calories per tablespoon), and a hands-down perfect substitute for high-fat dips and spreads. Salsa also contains lycopene, an antioxidant that may help prevent cancer, and it has absolutely no fat and only trace amounts of sodium.

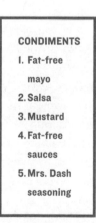

CONDIMENTS
1. Fat-free mayo
2. Salsa
3. Mustard
4. Fat-free sauces
5. Mrs. Dash seasoning

What I like most about salsa is that it has a zing that gives a kick to chili, soups, salads, or any other meal. Most salsas on the grocery store shelves are low calorie and low-fat. But shop wisely. You should still read the labels because a few of them have added sugar and higher calorie counts than you would expect. Avoid these at all costs!

My top picks: Pace salsas and Newman's Own salsas

3. Mustard. Mustard has three qualities that make it an ideal food: It adds consistency when mixed with other foods, it has a definite taste, and it's fat-free. (Stay away from mustards like honey mustard and Dijonnaise, which have more sugar and excess fat.) Whether you like it hot, spicy, regular, or yellow, mustard adds a sour or sweet spike, giving blander foods a bit of a kick.

My top pick: Gulden's Spicy Brown Mustard

4. Fat-free sauces. There are plenty of tasty sauces to choose from, but here are three that I highly recommend: soy, Worcestershire, and Tabasco. These are head and shoulders above the rest because they are practically calorie free—with no fat and no sugar—yet each packs a huge punch when it comes to adding tang, color, and flavor to foods. I find Worcestershire is an amazing sauce to perk up the flavor of soup as well as animal protein such as chicken or fish.

I'm not too concerned about whether you use a regular or low-sodium soy or Worcestershire sauce because most of the 5-Factor Must-Have Foods are low in sodium. Choose whichever one you think flavors your foods better.

If Tabasco is too intense for you, consider this: Research has shown that hot foods can mildly increase your metabolism. At the very least, a splash of Tabasco will encourage you to drink more water and fill up your belly even faster.

My top picks: 365 Organic Everyday Value Soy Ginger Sauce from Whole Foods Market and Lea & Perrins Worcestershire Sauce

5. Mrs. Dash. Why do I prefer this tried-and-true, sodium-free, sugar-free spice over all the other seasonings on the market? I'm not opposed to other brands, but I love that Mrs. Dash Seasoning Blend works with almost any food, making it the most versatile product I have in my kitchen. From fish and chicken to vegetables and soups, it's a great combination of herbs that turns even an amateur cook into a great chef. If you're not sure how to season something, just throw some Mrs. Dash on it and I guarantee it will taste terrific.

My top picks: The Mrs. Dash Original Blend is tasty, and it also comes in delicious flavors like Tomato Basil Garlic, Onion & Herb, Southwest Chipotle, and Extra Spicy. Include a few in your spice rack and you'll be ready to flavor up any meal.

SNACKS
1. Jerky. This superlean snack never needs to be refrigerated, so you can eat

and transport it anywhere. Jerky is usually made with high-quality animal protein and very little fat or carbohydrates. With all the fat stripped out, you're left with pure, muscle-building protein—and no worries about the calories.

Because jerky is a cured meat, it can be high in sodium. I'm not too concerned about the sodium levels, given that most of the foods in the 5-Factor Diet are naturally low in sodium. (If you're concerned about your sodium intake, drink plenty of water each time you eat jerky.) However, you should watch out for sugar. Some brands use it to make their jerky sweet; you'll find it in barbecue-flavored jerky, for example. Stick with the regular-flavor varieties or others without excess sugar.

My top picks: Ostrim Ostrich Meat Sticks, Pemmican Turkey Jerky, and Pioneer Turkey Jerky

2. Oatmeal. A bowl of oats can help you maintain an even level of energy throughout the day, according to research from Penn State University. That's because oats are loaded with extra soluble fiber, which slows down the release of sugar into the bloodstream.

> **SNACKS**
>
> 1. Jerky
> 2. Oatmeal
> 3. Ready to
>   Drinks (RTD)
> 4. Veggie
>   meats
> 5. Non-flour
>   crackers

I prefer to buy boxes of individual-serving oatmeal packets so I can take and make it anywhere with just a little hot water. Read the labels if you're shopping for flavored oatmeal; it often has added sugar, which defeats the purpose of eating it. Look for flavored versions that are either sugar free or low in sugar.

My top picks: Quick Quaker Oats and Quaker Weight Control oatmeal, which has fiber and protein added, comes in flavors like apple-cinnamon and banana and is very low in sugar.

3. RTDs (Ready to Drinks). RTDs are meal replacement drinks that come in convenient cans and drink boxes or in a mixable powder form. Essentially RTDs are complete meals in liquid form, fortified with vitamins, minerals, and enough calories to help sustain you. They can be as filling as an average meal, thanks to a great mix of protein, carbohydrates, and fat. The only thing missing typically is fiber, which is why I tell people to consume a fruit or a fiber cracker when having an RTD.

A very important point to remember is that RTDs are not a "liquid diet." In "Fad Diets Don't Work," page 12, I told you that liquid diets—in which you typically substitute shakes for meals—fail mostly because the drinks are basically water with just enough sugar to keep you barely functioning. RTDs are completely different. I think they're perfect, especially as an on-the-go snack, but certainly not as a replacement for several meals in a row.

My top picks: Lean Body Ready-to-Drink Shakes or RTDs from Met-Rx and Myoplex

4. Veggie Meats. Veggie dogs, veggie burgers, veggie bologna—today's grocery stores sell a wide assortment of faux meat products. They're smart substitutes for the real things because they contain very little fat, are typically as high in protein as real meat, and are extremely low in carbohydrates. They are also ideal to keep on hand in your fridge because they stay fresh as long as a month, which is a lot longer than fresh chicken, beef, or fish. If you doubt that they'll satisfy your taste buds, trust me when I say that food manufacturers have finally perfected the art of turning vegetables into a food that has all the flavor of real meat.

It's worth remembering that vegetarian meat isn't always healthier than regular meat. Certain brands of veggie burgers and veggie dogs are much higher in fat than I prefer. I suggest that you stick to products that are high in protein and get less than 20 percent of their calories from fat.

My top pick: Yves Veggie Cuisine products

5. No-flour Crackers and Brown Rice Cakes. No-flour crackers, made with whole grains instead of flour have roughly 5 grams of healthy fiber and less than 2 grams of fat per serving. Brown rice cakes are fat-free. These low-fat snacks are what I call the perfect "transport mechanism" for protein. Stack some turkey or smoked salmon on top and you'll get a high-protein, low-glycemic snack with a great crunch.

You'll find no-flour crackers and brown rice cakes in the health food section of your supermarket or right next to the less-healthy, flour-packed crackers and regular rice cakes.

When buying non-flour crackers, always check the list of ingredients on the package. You shouldn't find the word *flour* in any form—no flour, rice flour, wheat flour, rye flour, etc. Also look for the word *oil*. If you can find a brand with neither flour nor oil, you have a winner.

My top picks: Bran-a-crisp crackers, Quaker Rice Cakes (regular size)

5-FACTOR MUST-HAVE FOODS SHOPPING CHECKLIST

These are my celebrity clients' go-to foods. Now they're all yours. To be sure that you always have these 25 essential foods in your kitchen, copy this page and post it on your fridge. Shop so that you have at least one week's worth of each item in your home at all times.

PROTEINS

☐ Egg Whites

☐ Poultry

☐ Seafood

☐ Dairy

☐ Game

CONDIMENTS

☐ Fat-Free Mayo

☐ Salsa

☐ Mustard

☐ Fat-Free Sauces

☐ Mrs. Dash

CARBS

☐ Beans

☐ Grains

☐ Breads

☐ Vegetables

☐ Fruit

SNACKS

☐ Jerky

☐ Oatmeal Packets

☐ Ready To Drinks (RTDs)

☐ Veggie Meats

☐ No-flour Crackers

SUGAR-FREE BEVERAGES

☐ Water

☐ Coffee

☐ Tea

☐ Sugar-Free Juice

☐ Sugar-Free Soda

CHAPTER 8

Shopping for 5-Factor Foods

One of the greatest challenges of following any diet program is figuring out exactly how to incorporate it into your personal day-to-day routine. In this chapter, I'm going to show you how seamless the transition to a healthy lifestyle can be. An important part of this is rethinking your relationship with your grocery store. Being a smarter, savvier, healthier shopper just takes a little understanding about all the foods vying for your attention.

SMART WAYS TO NAVIGATE A GROCERY STORE

Sticking to the 5-Factor Diet requires you to make healthy choices, but that's not always easy to do when visiting the supermarket. How you shop and where you shop play a big role in whether you'll cheat on your diet. Use my 5-Factor shopping rules to ensure that every trip to the market is a healthy one.

1. SHOP EARLY

Even if you're not a morning person, make an effort to do your grocery shopping early in the day. Your body will thank you for it. Getting to the market early offers more than just avoiding the late-afternoon crowd—you'll also have your pick of the freshest foods available because most markets set out their produce and fresh meats in the morning. You can pick the best cuts of meat and choicest fruits and vegetables, thereby increasing your odds of choosing foods that are still packed with nutrients. Shop later in the day and you'll be stuck with older foods that have been picked through and, most likely, have lost nutrients.

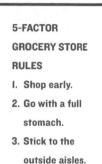

5-FACTOR GROCERY STORE RULES

1. Shop early.
2. Go with a full stomach.
3. Stick to the outside aisles.
4. Always have a plan.
5. Shop at the same store.

2. GO WITH A FULL STOMACH

Shopping for food when you're hungry is a recipe for disaster because your body desperately craves anything to fill its void, preferably something high in sugar and fat. That's why you should shop right after your first meal (breakfast) or your second meal (midmorning snack). That way, you'll feel satiated and be less tempted to pick up foods that aren't good for you.

3. STICK TO THE OUTSIDE AISLES

Most grocery stores share similar layouts, keeping their most healthy and nutritious foods around the perimeter. Do a lap around the store—going in one big rectangle—and you'll likely find almost all the foods on the 5-Factor Diet, including your produce, dairy, and meats. Avoid the inside aisles as much as possible; this is where you'll find most of the foods that are higher in fat and lower in nutrients. The only exception to this rule is the frozen food aisle, which is usually not on the perimeter. This is one of my favorite aisles when shopping for the 5-Factor Diet. (See "The Frozen Food Aisle is A Dieter's Best Friend," page 66.)

4. ALWAYS HAVE A PLAN

Never go to the supermarket without a well-thought-out list. Without a clear plan, you're more likely to buy bad foods on impulse. You may also forget to buy enough 5-Factor Foods. Remember, you need to eat foods from all five 5-Factor categories at each meal in order to achieve the best results, so missing even one of the five will hold back your progress.

I know you're busy, so simply copy the "5-Factor Must-Have Foods Shopping Checklist" on page 63 and you'll guarantee that you always have the right 5-Factor Diet foods in your kitchen.

5. SHOP AT THE SAME STORE

Once you find a store that carries all of the 5-Factor Diet foods, avoid frustration and shop only at that one store whenever possible. Being familiar with the layout of a store makes it much easier to get what you need quickly and avoid the aisles with bad foods. If you're regularly popping into unfamiliar supermarkets, you'll increase your risk of getting lost and walking past unhealthy goodies that may tempt you.

THE FROZEN FOOD AISLE IS A DIETER'S BEST FRIEND

Most dieters shy away from the frozen food aisle—and why wouldn't they? It's home to some of the most tempting, fattening foods around, from ice cream and frozen pizzas to those man-size TV dinners whose packaging has more nutrients than the actual food inside. If dieters do venture into this aisle, they probably zip past all the frozen desserts en route to the packaged—and pricey—diet meals put out by Healthy Choice and Weight Watchers. If this sounds like you, then you're missing out on all the great things the frozen food aisle has to offer—especially when it comes to implementing the 5-Factor Diet.

Every food has some sort of nutritional value, but its protein, vitamins, and minerals have a shelf life. From the moment a food is picked, caught, or killed, a nutritional clock starts ticking. Everything that happens to the food from that point forward ages it, affecting how much nutritional value you'll get from it when it finally finds its way to your mouth. As more people handle the food, the risk of it being tainted by things like bacteria or viruses increases. Every person that touches the food causes more bruising, which can make it spoil faster. The longer a food sits in a box or on a truck, the more it deteriorates. Even exposure to sunlight can degrade some of the important nutrients.

That's why the frozen food aisle is the 5-Factor dieter's greatest ally. Here are my top five reasons why you should no longer fear the frozen food aisle.

1. YOU GET MORE NUTRIENTS

When you buy frozen foods such as fruits and vegetables, they are flash-frozen almost immediately after they're harvested, so fewer people handle them. They're usually sealed in packages that are impervious to light. Time essentially stops, leaving all of the foods' nutrients sealed inside.

This means that when you buy a frozen strawberry at the grocery store, it's as nutritionally fresh as the day it was picked. After a good thaw, it is young and delicious again. On the other hand, a fresh strawberry in the produce aisle has an unknown history. It may have been picked out of state, then sifted, sorted, crated, warehoused, packaged, and trucked to a distribution center before being delivered to your local grocer and put out for display. It may have sat for as long as 10 days being touched by strangers and exposed to light. By the time you eat it, that strawberry is old. In fact, the FDA and the USDA have compared many fresh fruits and vegetables against frozen versions and found the two have relatively equivalent nutrient profiles. In fact, in some cases, certain nutrient levels are higher in the frozen foods.

> **BENEFITS OF FROZEN FOOD**
> 1. You get more nutrients.
> 2. It's convenient.
> 3. You'll save money.
> 4. It offers great variety.
> 5. You'll always have more healthy food around.

2. IT'S CONVENIENT

I love raw vegetables, but sometimes a bag of frozen mixed veggies or stir-fry veggies is more convenient. Fresh vegetables require a lot of cleaning and chopping. With frozen veggies, all that hard work has been done for you. Just grab a bag of mixed vegetables and they're ready to be added to a stir-fry or made into a side dish. Frozen meats and fish are even more of a time-saver. With no cleaning involved, just thaw and you're ready to cook—mess free!

3. YOU'LL SAVE MONEY

A lot of my clients think frozen foods are more expensive, but ask yourself this: How many times have you thrown away fresh chicken, fish, fruits, or vegetables because they sat around in your fridge too long? We've all done it. With frozen foods, you rarely have to throw anything away because it has spoiled; most foods stay fresh for months in the freezer.

4. IT OFFERS GREAT VARIETY

I'm big on berries, but they aren't in season as often as I'd like. Luckily, I can always find them in the frozen food aisle, along with any other out-of-season fruits I may be craving.

I recommend you keep a big bag of stir-fry vegetables in the freezer. Why? Because a lot of dieters stick with eating the same veggies over and over again. Don't get me wrong; eating vegetables is good, but different vegetables often have different amounts of vitamins and minerals. If you're eating the same one or two vegetables, you may be getting a lot of, say, vitamin A while missing out on iron or vitamin C. Eating a handful of stir-fry veggies (I like to steam them) gives you an assortment every time, so you're guaranteed a balanced mix of nutrients.

5. YOU'LL ALWAYS HAVE HEALTHY FOOD AROUND

Having lots of healthy food around is terrific, but it's not always practical to buy a 10-pound tray of fresh chicken breasts from the meat department! But you can find these foods in the frozen aisle, along with fruits and vegetables that come in 5- to 10-pound bags. Buying in bulk may seem like a space eater in your freezer, but it works to your advantage. It guarantees that you'll always have healthy foods to eat (and less space

---

TIPS FOR BUYING FROZEN FOODS

1. Buy vegetables raw—and never with cheese sauce or butter packets!

2. Before buying fruit, read the label. The only ingredient should be the fruit itself, not syrup.

3. When you pick up meat, gently squeeze the package. If you hear or feel a crunch, it's probably freezer-burned.

4. Always reach into the back of the freezer, where food is kept colder.

5. Read the cooking instructions. Some frozen foods are precooked, which means you could be getting more sugars and bad fats than if they were raw.

to stock unhealthy options). By keeping the freezer well stocked, you'll never run out and be left reaching for something off the 5-Factor Diet when you're hungry.

PICKING THE BEST SWEETENERS

When you shop for healthy foods, you'll come across many low- or reduced-calorie foods. They may sound good, but it's important to know exactly what natural or artificial substitute you're eating in place of sugar. Some of these sweeteners may be great for adding calorie-free flavor to your food, but many come with health issues of which you should be aware.

THE SEVEN MOST COMMON SUGAR SUBSTITUTES

I have to break from my use of the number 5 for a moment because we need to examine seven common sweeteners used today: sucrose, turbinado, honey, aspartame, saccharin, sucralose (Splenda), and stevia. You should make your own personal decision about which sweeteners to use, based on the facts about these products, including what the manufacturers won't tell you. Here's the truth—and my recommendations—about sweeteners.

> "My biggest problem was finding a diet that accommodated my busy schedule. Between work, travel, and my family, I had no time to get in shape. Your diet was so simple to follow, with suitable food choices and simple substitutions. The rapid changes I experienced only increased my motivation to succeed. Thank you!"
>
> **David Widman, M.D.** AGE: 41 WEIGHT LOST: 15 lbs. in 4 weeks

Sucrose (or sugar). Sucrose is the most common food sweetener in the world. Extracted from sugar cane or sugar beets, it's purified and crystallized, then stripped of all vitamins, minerals, fiber, amino acids, and trace elements. It may be nutritionally worthless, but because of its taste and the quick hit of energy it provides, sugar is a hard habit to kick.

Unfortunately, the fleeting burst of energy usually disappears as quickly as it came, leaving you feeling more sluggish than you did before eating. This effect is called "reactive hypoglycemia." Think of it this way: Eating sugar is like accelerating your car by flooring the gas, then taking your foot off the pedal and letting the car go back to its normal speed. At a certain point, your car will slow down to the speed at which it was running before you hit the gas, then slow down even further (and eventually stop altogether). When you eat sugar, your energy levels ultimately dip below your baseline, which is why you end up craving even more sugar later.

It's a vicious cycle, and it's the reason why we obsess about sweet foods. But our consumption comes at a price. Just like highly glycemic carbohydrates, sugar causes an insulin surge that makes your body store calories as fat—even if you're eating fat-free sweets. Research has shown that sugar has the same effect as other carbohydrates on blood sugar levels. Calorie for calorie, sugar raises blood glucose about the same amount as starches such as white bread and white potatoes.

Turbinado. You may not recognize its real name, but you've seen it in the light brown packets. It's that dark brown, coarse, "raw" sugar that's supposed to be better for you because it's all-natural and chemical free. (White table sugar, by comparison, is processed with things like phosphoric acid, sulphur dioxide, and bleaching agents, to name just a few!) Turbinado is usually made by squeezing the juice out of crushed sugar cane, then spinning what's left after evaporation through a huge centrifuge. Because it's not chemically treated, it's supposed to be richer in vitamins and minerals.

Wrong! The big mistake most people make is assuming that turbinado is healthier than table sugar because it's unbleached. This assumption causes some people to use even more of it than they would regular sugar. People make a similar mistake when comparing white bread with breads that are dyed brown to seem more natural. But just because something is darker doesn't always mean it's better for you! White sugar and dark sugar may have different characteristics and tastes, but your body reacts to both in the same way, with a fat-storing insulin spike.

Honey. I don't recommend honey. Honey producers make a lot of healthy promises, claiming honey can protect you against cancer and heart disease because it contains antioxidants and certain enzymes. The problem is, honey—no matter how unrefined and all-natural its producers may say it is—is still nothing more than pure sugar. To be exact, it's an invert sugar—created by an enzyme in bee nectar—that's an extremely dense, gelatinous form of easily absorbed sugar. At best, honey has only trace amounts of antioxidants, vitamins, and minerals. That's true whether you're talking about buckwheat honey, sunflower honey, or regular clover honey.

Honey should never take the place of fruits and veggies, which are far richer in antioxidants and have much less sugar. You get far more antioxidants and nutrients from a single piece of fruit than you ever could from pouring on honey and adding excess sugar to your diet. It's the wrong approach.

Aspartame. You may know it by other names (such as NutraSweet or Equal), but aspartame is a low-calorie sweetener that is about 200 times sweeter than sugar. However, it's not the best sweetener for use in hot drinks or cooking because it tends to lose its sweetness in high temperatures. That's why coffee or tea drinkers who use aspartame may find themselves pouring in extra packets when reaching for their morning pick-me-up.

There is a great deal of controversy over this sweetener, especially because it's made from methyl alcohol, which on its own is potentially toxic. Despite that, aspartame has been proven safe for human consumption. However, people with a rare hereditary metabolic condition called phenylketonuria (PKU) need to watch their intake of aspartame because it contains the enzyme phenylalanine, which they must avoid. That's why some product labels print "This product contains phenylalanine" on them. If you're pregnant, avoid aspartame because it's impossible to know if your baby has PKU.

Personally, I don't like the taste of aspartame but if you want to use it, I would prefer that you have it in small amounts only.

WHAT IS "PERCENT DAILY VALUE"?

Understanding Percent Daily Values—which is often shortened to "% Daily Value" or "%DV"—is key to deciphering any food label. These percentages tell you how a single serving of the food fits into a typical 2,000-calorie-a-day meal plan. (If you consume more or less than 2,000 calories, you need to adjust the Percent Daily Value accordingly.) At a glance, you can tell whether a food is high or low in a specific nutrient. For example, the label might tell you that a food provides 13% of your recommended daily value of carbohydrates or 35% of your fats. It's also a snap to compare the nutrients in products against each other—just be sure the serving sizes match first.

Sugars, protein, and trans fats don't have a Percent Daily Value, so you won't see a percentage listed for them. The FDA hasn't determined yet how much protein the average person should consume daily. As for sugar and trans fats, the FDA doesn't want you eating either, so it naturally doesn't recommend any set amount.

Saccharin. Sweet'N Low and Sugar Twin are two brands of saccharin you're most likely familiar with. Saccharin is so popular because it can sweeten both hot and cold foods and is low calorie. Some people have had concerns about the sweetener because older studies found that rats who ingested large amounts of the sweetener were at risk for cancer. New research has found saccharin is safe in the small amounts most people use. But I'll be honest with you—I'm not a big saccharin fan. In fact, following a 1977 study in which rats got bladder cancer after being fed saccharin, Canada, where I am originally from, banned it from being sold. It still is not sold there, which should say something in itself. If you choose to use saccharin in lieu of sugar, I recommend the smallest amounts possible, just to be safe.

Stevia. Stevia is a natural dietary supplement extracted from the *Stevia rebaudiana* plant, and it has been used for decades around the world, especially in Japan. It's about 300 times sweeter than sugar and is calorie-free. Go to any health food store and you'll see it touted as the most popular natural alternative to sugar. However, the FDA hasn't approved it for use as a sweetener. Why not? A few studies have shown that stevia may cause cancer and reproductive health problems, which is why Canada and some other countries won't allow it to be used as a sweetener. The FDA does state that when used sparingly, stevia is perfectly safe—although the agency believes it could create health issues if approved as an artificial sweetener. Stevia is definitely an acquired taste; it can change the flavor of foods and beverages.

Sucralose (Splenda). Sucralose is 600 times sweeter than sugar and the newest low-calorie sweetener on the market—and is my sweetener of choice. It's basically regular table sugar that's been chlorinated, a process that tweaks it just enough so that it doesn't make your blood sugar rise. It also retains its sweetness in hot and cold foods.

To this point, there haven't been any negative findings in research on sucralose usage. In Canada, we've been using it for about 15 years.

DECIPHERING FOOD LABELS

Before I start working with clients, I give them reading material about nutrition. We talk everything through and I teach them how to cook, whether they want to or not. If they want to taste my food, they have to watch me cook it. Why? Because I want to empower them. Once they understand how their bodies work with the foods they eat, following the 5-Factor Diet is even easier. They gain a sense of confidence in the program, even when I'm not there. They can follow my advice without having to question why it works.

WHAT TO EXPECT ON A FOOD LABEL

SERVING SIZE

SERVINGS PER CONTAINER

CALORIES

  Calories from fat

TOTAL FAT

  Saturated fat

  Trans fat

  Polyunsaturated fat

  Monounsaturated fat

CHOLESTEROL

SODIUM

TOTAL CARBOHYDRATES

  Dietary fiber

  Sugars

  Other carbohydrates

PROTEIN

VITAMINS AND MINERALS

  Vitamin A

  Vitamin C

  Calcium

  Iron

  Vitamin D

  Thiamin

  Riboflavin

  Niacin

  Vitamin B$_6$

  Phosphorus

  Magnesium

  Zinc

LESS THAN SERIES

LIST OF INGREDIENTS

A lot of diet books tell you what to eat and maybe a little bit about why you should eat that way. But they don't empower you to make good choices for yourself. Being able to decipher what's in every single food gives you power. You can finally look through your fridge and cupboards and understand—maybe for the first time in your life—what will work and what won't work for your diet.

WHAT YOU NEED TO KNOW

In this book you're already learning the science of nutrition. How you apply that knowledge starts with understanding the foods you eat. That's why knowing how to read a nutritional label is one of the most important lessons I can teach you. Here's the information you'll find on the label— and what those numbers mean to you.

Serving size. This number tells you what quantity of the food was used to determine the nutrition facts. To make it easy for you to compare it to other, similar foods, the measurements are usually standard: The label will first list the serving size in lay terms (such as ½ cup or 6 pieces), then give you the metric amount (122 grams, for example).

5-Factor Fact: Most people eat a lot more than the recommended serving size. Try portioning out one serving size to get a better sense of how many servings you're really eating when you have that food.

Servings per container. This number tells you the approximate number of servings the package contains.

5-Factor Fact: This information is amazingly helpful. Some foods have very small serving sizes so that the amount of calories per serving seems low. That is, until you do the math. Multiplying the "servings per container" by "calories per serving" will give you the caloric content of the entire package.

Calories and calories from fat. In addition to telling you how many calories you're getting per serving, the label also shows exactly how many of those calories are from fat.

5-Factor Fact: Seeing big numbers in the "calories from fat" section shouldn't always scare you. Good-for-you fats such as olive oil get *all* of their calories from fat.

Total fat. This number combines the fat grams from all four types of fats: saturated, trans, polyunsaturated, and monounsaturated.

5-Factor Fact: The FDA suggests that you eat no more than 65 grams of fat per day.

Saturated fat. This is the number of saturated fat grams contained in each serving.

5-Factor Fact: Your daily maximum of this unhealthy fat is 20 grams, according to the FDA. I suggest keeping your intake of this dangerous fat even lower.

Trans fat. This shows how many grams of trans fat are in each serving.

5-Factor Fact: In January 2006, the FDA began requiring all food manufacturers to list trans fat on their labels. That's good news because

---

Alicia Keys GRAMMY-WINNING SINGER/SONGWRITER

"Harley's style of working out is 100 percent my style. It doesn't take a lot of time out of your day, it's motivating, and you feel good (especially when people take notice!). The focus is not on starving yourself but on healthful living, so you don't feel like you're missing out on the foods you love. Once you get started, you get addicted to looking, feeling, and living your best."

GOOD NEWS FOR ALLERGY SUFFERERS

Each year approximately 30,000 people in the United States require emergency room treatment and 150 die because of allergic reactions to food. Now, new food label laws may help prevent some of these problems. In January I, 2006, the FDA began requiring that food labels clearly identify when ingredients contain protein derived from the eight major allergenic foods: milk, eggs, fish, crustacean shellfish, tree nuts, peanuts, wheat, and soybeans. If you're allergic to these foods, read the list of ingredients; you should find any troublesome ingredient listed along with the source of the food allergen.

---

before this it was tough to determine what foods contained this dangerous form of fat. Don't expect to find a Percent Daily Value listed for this bad-for-you fat, because your body doesn't need it. Keep your consumption of trans fat as close to zero as possible.

Polyunsaturated fat. This is the total number of polyunsaturated fat grams per serving.

5-Factor Fact: Unlike saturated fat, polyunsaturated fat doesn't raise cholesterol levels. Rather, it actually lowers the amount of bad cholesterol lipids, called low-density lipoproteins (LDLs).

Monounsaturated fat. This is the total number of monounsaturated fat grams in each serving.

5-Factor Fact: Olive oil is an excellent source of monounsaturated fat, plus it makes a great base for salad dressing.

Cholesterol. This is the total milligrams of cholesterol per serving.

5-Factor Fact: Although your body needs cholesterol to assist with hormone production and other bodily functions, your liver manufactures cholesterol on its own. That's why you should limit your daily intake to 300 milligrams.

Sodium. This is the total milligrams of sodium per serving.

5-Factor Fact: I'm not overly concerned about excess sodium in the diet because only a very small percentage of the population is sodium sensitive. Sodium is relatively benign and passes out of the body

"For me, starting a new program was less about losing a bunch of weight and more about wanting to finally tone and shape my middle-age body. My butt and thighs were beginning to make a world of their own! I didn't understand which foods were beneficial and which ones should simply be avoided, but the nutrition explanations in 5-Factor taught me what I should aim for with each and every meal."

Mashell Smith AGE: **44** WEIGHT LOST SO FAR: **7 lbs.**

fairly quickly. The FDA recommends keeping your daily intake below 2,400 milligrams. Of course, if you have high blood pressure or kidney issues, then you should monitor your sodium intake more closely.

Total carbohydrates. This number is the total grams of every type of carbohydrate—dietary fiber, sugars, and other sources—per serving.

5-Factor Fact: The FDA suggests a daily total carb consumption of 300 grams or less. As you already know, I want you to eat only carbs with low to moderate glycemic levels. But food labels don't tell you what the carbohydrates' glycemic level is. To find out, go to the glycemic index database at www.glycemicindex.com.

Dietary fiber. This is how many grams of fiber—both soluble and insoluble—are in each serving. This amount is included in the total carbohydrates measurement, but dietary fiber affects blood sugar less than other types of carbs do. That's why the American Diabetes Association suggests that if a food has 5 grams or more of fiber per serving, you can subtract this number from the carbohydrate total.

5-Factor Fact: Fiber comes in two types—soluble and insoluble—but nutrition labels aren't required to list them separately. However, most manufacturers will tell you somewhere on the package how many grams of insoluble fiber their product contains.

Sugars. This is where you'll see how many grams of sugar are in each serving. You may also see "sugar alcohols" or "sugar replacers" listed. Sugar alcohols don't affect your blood sugar levels as much as sugar does, but they have a caloric value 10 percent greater than other carbs.

5-Factor Fact: If you see grams of sugar on the nutrition label but can't find the word *sugar* on the list of ingredients, that's because sugar sometimes goes by different names. Check the list for names like fructose (fruit sugar), glucose (dextrose), galactose (milk sugar), lactose (a combination of glucose and galactose), and maltose (malt sugar).

Other carbohydrates. This number—which isn't on all labels—is a catch-all category for any other types of carbohydrates that may be in each serving.

5-Factor Fact: These trace carbs—typically various organic acids and flavenoids—don't raise your blood sugar level very much, so don't be concerned about them. Sometimes sugar alcohols are thrown into this category as well; sugar alcohols may include malitol, sorbitol, xylitol, and glycerine.

Protein. This is how many grams of protein are in each serving.

5-Factor Fact: Sometimes dairy protein appears on an ingredient list in the form of albumen, whey, or casein.

Vitamin and mineral percentages. All food labels are required to list vitamin A, vitamin C, calcium, and iron content. Other nutrients—such as vitamin D, thiamin, riboflavin, niacin, vitamin B6, phosphorus, magnesium, and zinc—are shown only if they're added as a supplement.

You won't see how many grams or milligrams of each nutrient are in a serving. Instead you'll see what percentage of the recommended daily amount of that nutrient is contained in each serving.

Ingredients. Finally, a label lists all the food's ingredients, arranged in descending order based on the weight of each ingredient.

5-Factor Fact: Because of the ranking of ingredients by weight, the first few ingredients listed are typically the bulk of what's in the food. For a real eye-opener, compare the ingredients list of a processed food with its natural equivalent—for instance, processed, sugary fruit drink versus 100 percent fresh-squeezed juice. The differences will startle you.

Tracee Ross ACTRESS AND STAR ON THE TV SHOW *GIRLFRIENDS*

"Harley has taught me to love my body in a way I haven't since I was 18. I just want to run around naked with a tattoo on my ass that says, "Body by Harley." Harley has taught me how to keep myself toned, lean, and strong and still have that perfect amount of womanly jiggle so I look and feel good on and off screen. Since I met Harley, I am never more than two weeks from my ideal."

LEARN THE LINGO

If you see this word ...	Then the food contains ...
LEAN	Less than I0 grams of fat, 4 grams of saturated fat, and 95 milligrams of cholesterol.
EXTRA LEAN	Less than 5 grams of fat, 2 grams of saturated fat, and 95 milligrams of cholesterol.
REDUCED FAT	25% less fat than the regular version.
MORE	At least I0% more of a specific nutrient, compared to the regular version.
GOOD SOURCE OF	I0–I9% of the Daily Value of a particular nutrient.
HIGH IN	20% or more of the Daily Value recommended for that particular nutrient.
LIGHT OR LITE	At least one-third fewer calories than the regular version of that food, or no more than half of the fat. If you see the word in reference to sodium, it means the food has at least 50% less sodium than the regular version.

If you see this word ...	Then the food contains ...

LOW	Less of a particular nutrient per serving than the regular version of that food. How much less depends on the nutrient.
	    If a food is "low calorie," it has less than 40 calories per serving.
	    If a food is "low fat," it has less than 3 grams of total fat per serving.
	    If a food is "low in saturated fat," it has less than I gram of saturated fat per serving.
	    If a food is "low cholesterol," it has less than 20 milligrams of cholesterol per serving.
	    If a food is "low sodium," it has less than I40 milligrams of sodium per serving.
	    If a food is "very low sodium," it has less than 35 milligrams per serving.

FREE	Little or no trace of a particular nutrient per serving.
	    If a food is "calorie-free," it has less than 5 calories per serving.
	    If a food is "fat-free" it has less than 0.5 gram of total fat per serving.
	    If a food is "free of saturated fat," it has less than 0.5 gram of saturated fat per serving.
	    If a food is "cholesterol-free," it has less than 2 milligrams of cholesterol per serving.
	    If a food is "sodium-free," it has less than 5 milligrams of sodium per serving.
	    If a food is "sugar-free," it has less than 0.5 gram of sugars per serving.

% FAT-FREE	This designates the actual amount of a food that is not made up of fat. But don't be fooled. A product may be "90% fat-free," but the other I0% might be loaded in calories.
REDUCED	At least 25% less of a nutrient, compared to the regular product.

CHAPTER 9

New 5-Factor Hollywood Workout

You can't transform your body through diet alone.

Burning fat, shaping your muscles, feeling better, and being healthier—it all starts with a smart eating plan and an equally smart exercise program. Other diets "suggest" exercise without giving specifics, or they prescribe a regimen that's too complex or too time-consuming for anyone with a life. The 5-Factor program is not like any other diet you've ever tried.

My first book, *5-Factor Fitness*, focused more on exercise, while in this book I've been able to give you more nutritional information and exciting, delicious recipes to try. Still, exercise remains a major component of my program if you want the best results possible.

If you have my first book, you're in for a treat. The exercises and routines in this chapter are all new, yet equally effective, so you'll build even more lean muscle tissue and burn off even more body fat. I'll also show you how to extend the original five-week workout plan into a five-month fitness regime that will truly take your body to the next level. If you're brand-new to exercise and 5-Factor fitness, don't worry. My plan is the easiest, most effective exercise program you'll ever use.

5-FACTOR HOLLYWOOD WORKOUT SECRETS

The 5-Factor Hollywood Workout routine, just like my 5-Factor Diet, is simple: You'll do 5 workouts a week, each 25 minutes long and broken into the following five 5-minute phases:

Phase 1: 5 minutes of cardio warm-up
Phase 2: 5 minutes of upper-body strength training
Phase 3: 5 minutes of lower-body strength training
Phase 4: 5 minutes of core training
Phase 5: 5 minutes of fat-burning cardio work

That's it. If you can give me—or should I say, your body—125 minutes total of attention each week for a recommended five-week cycle, your results will amaze you.

With the 5-Factor Diet's 5-phase workout, I've had clients lose 5 or more pounds a month, without ever feeling like they're spending all their time working out. In fact, by tweaking the final cardio portion of the workout, you can burn off even more body fat, as I'll explain when I describe Phase 5 in detail.

I'm sure you're wondering how a workout that takes so little time can be so effective. You shouldn't be surprised that I have five very good reasons!

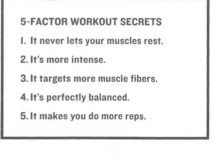

5-FACTOR WORKOUT SECRETS

1. It never lets your muscles rest.
2. It's more intense.
3. It targets more muscle fibers.
4. It's perfectly balanced.
5. It makes you do more reps.

1. IT NEVER LETS YOUR MUSCLES REST

The 5-Factor Hollywood Workout uses an advanced technique called "supersetting," in which you do two exercises back-to-back without resting in between. This makes the workout shorter but keeps your heart rate elevated longer, so you burn more calories.

2. IT'S MORE INTENSE

Most workout routines have you perform exercises exactly the same way every time. For instance, you may be asked to do three sets of 12 repetitions per exercise, with 60 seconds of rest between sets. The 5-Factor Workout, on the other hand, constantly changes the type of exercise, the number of repetitions, the rest time between super-sets, and the resistance level of your workout. Because the workout is constantly changing, your body never gets bored so it keeps evolving, keeps burning fat, and never stops progressing.

3. IT TARGETS MORE MUSCLE FIBERS

Many workouts you see in magazines string together exotic exercises that isolate only specific, small muscle groups. The problem with that approach? To burn the most calories, you have to involve as many muscles as possible.

That's why the 5-Factor Workout targets large muscle groups, such as your chest, back, quadriceps, and hamstrings, twice a week. Smaller muscle groups, such as your biceps, triceps, and shoulders, get a workout once a week.

4. IT'S PERFECTLY BALANCED

The muscles on the front of your body (chest, biceps, quadriceps) work in tandem with the muscles on the back of your body (back, triceps, and hamstrings). Most routines don't account for that fact, and they end up working one side of the body more than the other. With the 5-Factor Hollywood Workout, you work opposing muscle groups equally, so your body gets a balanced workout.

5. IT MAKES YOU DO MORE REPS

Other routines call for 8 to 12 repetitions of each exercise—or maybe go as high as 15. The 5-Factor Hollywood Workout pushes your muscles beyond average levels of fatigue by sometimes requiring 15 to 25 reps. This technique uses more calories, so you end up burning off even more body fat.

THE 5 PHASES OF THE 5-FACTOR HOLLYWOOD WORKOUT

My workout breaks down into 5 phases, each of which lasts for 5 minutes. You'll always start with Phase 1, then move to Phase 2, then Phase 3, then Phase 4, and finish with Phase 5. From start to finish, the routine takes only 25 minutes. To give your body a chance to recover, you'll exercise five days a week and incorporate a rest day twice a week. (In this book, I've made Wednesday and Sunday rest days; feel free to choose whichever two days are best for your schedule.) To get the best results, follow my 5-week program, which builds up intensity gradually so that by week 5, your body is burning calories at its highest possible pace.

PHASE 1: 5-MINUTE CARDIO WARM-UP
Warm up with 5 minutes of light cardio exercise. You can walk, cycle, stair climb, or use a cardio machine set on a low level. It doesn't matter what you do because the goal is just to get your blood flowing to warm up muscles, tendons, and joints.

> **5-FACTOR HOLLYWOOD WORKOUT**
> Phase 1: Cardio Warm-up
> Phase 2: Upper-Body Strength Training
> Phase 3: Lower-Body Strength Training
> Phase 4: Core Training
> Phase 5: Cardio Work

Begin at a low intensity. Gradually increase the intensity by speeding up the activity you're doing. By the end of the 5 minutes, I want your heart rate elevated so you're in a fat-burning zone when you start Phases 2 and 3.

As you warm up, check your pulse by placing two fingers either on the side of your neck or on the front of your wrist just below your palm. Count the heartbeats for 10 seconds, then multiply that number by 6 to determine your pulse rate in beats per minute (BPM). By the end of your warm-up, your BPM should fall within the appropriate range below to burn fat efficiently. (If your BPM is less than suggested, up your intensity in the next workout; if it's higher than suggested, lower your intensity in the next workout.)

Age	Pulse	Age	Pulse
20–24	130–170	55–59	107–140
25–29	127–166	60–64	104–136
30–34	124–162	65–69	101–132
35–39	120–157	70–74	98–128
40–44	117–153	75–79	94–123
45–49	114–149	80+	91–119
50–54	111–145		

PHASES 2 AND 3: 10 MINUTES OF STRENGTH TRAINING (UPPER AND LOWER BODY)

Phase 2 and Phase 3, which together work all of the upper- and lower-body muscles, are combined for a good reason—to keep your heart rate elevated so you burn fat as you build muscle.

For 10 minutes, you'll do two different exercises back-to-back, resting only after completing a superset made up of both exercises. Refer to the charts below to see how many repetitions to perform (it varies by week) and how many seconds to rest between supersets. Repeat this cycle for the prescribed number of supersets.

Here are the 10 exercises you'll use over the course of the week.

Day	Exercise	Core muscles involved
1: Monday	Incline Dumbbell Flys (upper body)	Chest
	Ball Wall Squats (lower body)	Quadriceps
2: Tuesday	Reverse Incline Dumbbell Rows (upper body)	Back
	Dumbbell Deadlifts (lower body)	Hamstrings
3: Wednesday	Off	
4: Thursday	Incline Dumbbell Bicep Curls (upper body)	Biceps
	Overhead Dumbbell Tricep Extensions (upper body)	Triceps
5: Friday	Dumbbell Lateral Raises (upper body)	Shoulders
	Step-Ups (lower body)	Quadriceps
6: Saturday	Bent-Over Dumbbell Rows (upper body)	Back
	Lying Ball Hamstring Curls (lower body)	Hamstrings
7: Sunday	Off	

If you're a beginner or intermediate exerciser, here's your plan!

Week	For each exercise	Rest after each superset
1	25 reps, 2 supersets,	80 seconds
2	20 reps, 3 supersets	70 seconds
3	15 reps, 3 supersets	60 seconds
4	16 reps, 4 supersets	50 seconds
5	10 reps, 5 supersets	40 seconds

If you're an advanced exerciser, here's your plan!

Week	For each exercise	Rest after each superset
1	30 reps, 3 supersets	90 seconds
2	25 reps, 3 supersets	70 seconds
3	20 reps, 4 supersets	50 seconds
4	15 reps, 4 supersets	40 seconds
5	12 reps, 5 supersets	30 seconds

As you see, you'll be varying the repetitions and adding more supersets as the weeks progress. The rest time between supersets also decreases each week. The exercises themselves stay the same throughout this 5-week plan.

THE ONLY EQUIPMENT YOU NEED

To do the 5-Factor Workout, all you need is a set of dumbbells, a bench with an incline feature (if you don't have one, modify the exercises as described), and a stability ball.

When using dumbbells, pick a weight that's heavy enough so you can just barely complete the prescribed repetitions with perfect form. For example, if an exercise calls for you to do 16 repetitions and you could have done 18, your dumbbell isn't heavy enough to work your muscles, and you're cheating yourself of results.

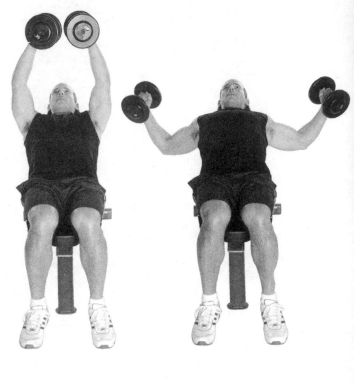

STRENGTH TRAINING EXERCISES
DAY 1: MONDAY

INCLINE DUMBBELL FLYS

Lie flat on your back on an incline bench with a dumbbell in each hand. Raise your arms above you so the weights come together directly above your chest, palms facing each other. Bend your elbows slightly and slowly lower your arms out to the sides until the weights are in line with your chest. Slowly sweep your arms back up until they are over your chest—imagine you're hugging a wide barrel—and repeat.

If you don't have an incline bench: Do this exercise while lying on a flat bench instead.

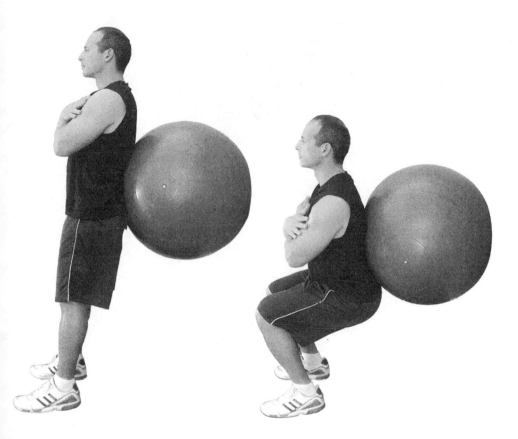

BALL WALL SQUATS

Stand a few feet away from a wall with your back toward the wall. Tuck a
stability ball between your back and the wall, then lean back against the
ball until your entire upper body is supported by the ball and the wall.
Maintaining your balance, cross your arms in front of your chest, then slowly
squat down until your thighs are parallel to the floor. The ball should roll
down the wall as you go. Slowly stand back up and repeat.

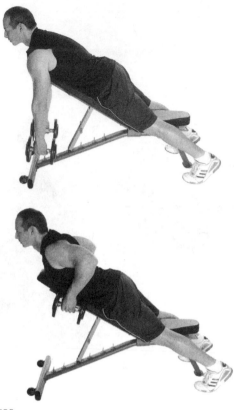

DAY 2: TUESDAY

REVERSE INCLINE DUMBBELL ROWS

Lie facedown on an incline bench, with your chest flat against the elevated pad. Hold a dumbbell in each hand, letting your arms hang down to the floor, palms facing each other. Keeping your chest on the bench and your arms close to your torso, pull both dumbbells up to the sides of your chest. Slowly lower your arms back down and repeat.

If you don't have an incline bench: You can do the exercise one arm at a time. Stand with your right side toward a bench—or bed—and a dumbbell in your left hand. Rest your right hand and knee on the bench, bend forward at the waist, and let your left arm hang down toward the floor. Slowly pull the weight up to the side of your chest, then lower it. Repeat with other arm.

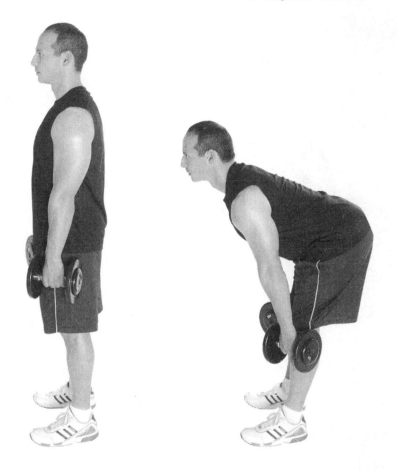

DUMBBELL DEADLIFTS

Position a dumbbell on the floor along the outside of each foot, then stand tall. Bend your knees and grasp the dumbbells with your palms facing in. Keeping your head up and your back straight, slowly stand up until your legs are straight, knees unlocked. Make sure the weights stay close to your body as you stand. Slowly reverse the motion and place the dumbbells back down on the floor. Repeat.

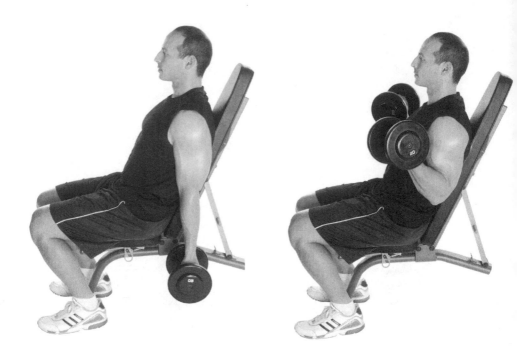

DAY 4: THURSDAY

INCLINE DUMBBELL BICEP CURLS

Lie faceup on an incline bench with a dumbbell in each hand, letting your arms hang straight down toward the floor. Your palms should face up toward the front. Keeping your upper arms stationary, slowly curl both weights up until they are in front of your chest—remember to curl both weights up at the same time. Slowly lower the weights back down and repeat.

If you don't have an incline bench: Do this exercise standing up instead.

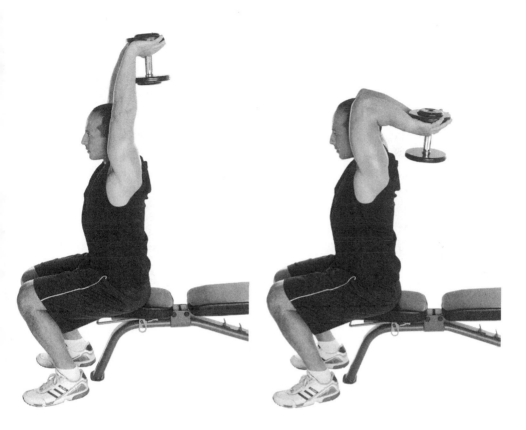

OVERHEAD DUMBBELL
TRICEP EXTENSIONS

Sit on a chair or an exercise bench with your back straight. Place your feet firmly on the floor and grasp a single dumbbell with both hands. Raise the weight above your head, rotating it so the top plate rests comfortably in the palms of your hands, with your thumbs around the handle. Slowly lower the weight behind your head until your forearms touch your biceps. Straighten your arms to raise the weight back over your head. Repeat.

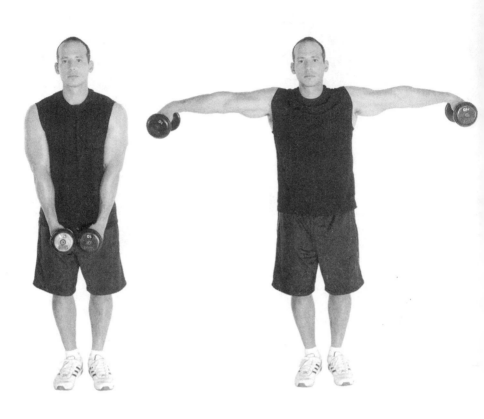

DAY 5: FRIDAY

DUMBBELL LATERAL RAISES

Stand with your arms in front of you with a dumbbell in each hand, palms facing each other. Keeping your arms straight and your wrists slightly bent, slowly raise the weights out to the sides until your arms are parallel to the floor (you'll look like the letter T). Pause for a second, then slowly lower your arms back down in front of you so the dumbbells touch each other right below your waistline. Repeat.

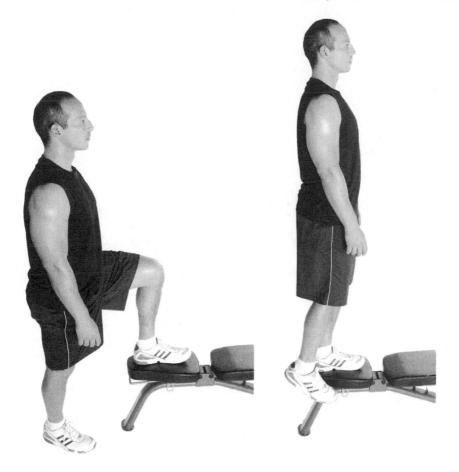

STEP-UPS

Stand in front of an exercise bench (or a sturdy box or staircase). Let your arms hang at your sides. With your back straight, place your left foot on the bench and push yourself up onto the bench until your left leg is straight. You don't have to bring your right foot onto the bench unless you need to balance yourself. Reverse the exercise by stepping back down and placing both feet back on the floor. Repeat the exercise, using the same leg, for the number of repetitions prescribed. Then change positions to work the opposite leg, this time placing your right foot on the bench.

For added intensity, you may do this exercise while holding a dumbbell in each hand.

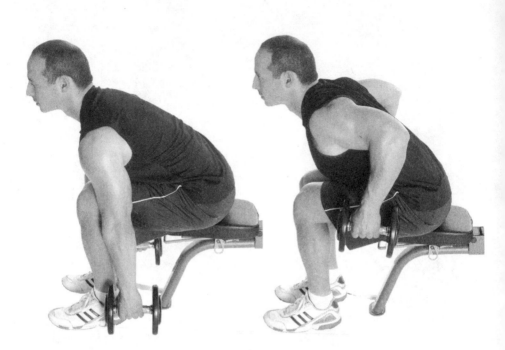

DAY 6: SATURDAY

BENT-OVER DUMBBELL ROWS

Sit on the edge of a bench holding a dumbbell in each hand. Bend forward at the waist—keeping your back flat—until your back is almost parallel to the floor (your chest should come down as close to your thighs as possible). Let your arms hang straight down, with palms facing each other. Slowly draw your elbows up as high as you can, keeping your arms close to your sides. Pause, then slowly lower them back down until your arms are straight once again. Repeat.

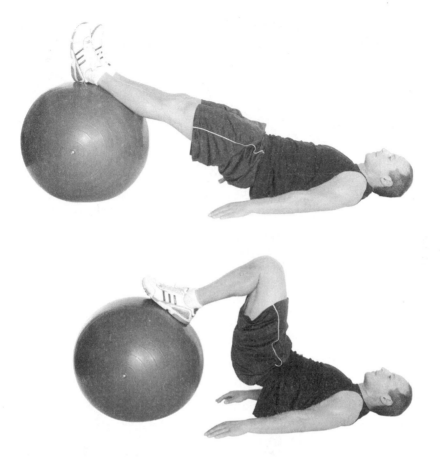

LYING BALL HAMSTRING CURLS

Lie flat on your back with your arms flat on the floor and your heels on top of a stability ball. Press your heels down onto the ball, then tighten your core muscles. Slowly raise your hips up and draw your heels—and the ball—toward your butt as far as you can. Pause, then roll the ball back by straightening your legs; your hips will naturally lower back to the floor as you reverse the motion. Repeat.

PHASE 4: 5 MINUTES OF CORE TRAINING
Phase 4 targets all four muscle groups that make up your core. You'll do
one abdominal exercise each day, but five different ones over the course
of the week. Days 1–4 each focus on one individual muscle group plus
the specific ab-toning move, and Day 5 works as many muscle groups as
possible in one single exercise.

Here's the plan:

Day	Exercise	Core muscles involved
1: Monday	Ball Crunches	Upper Rectus Abdominis
2: Tuesday	Seated Dumbbell Side Bends	Lateral Obliques
3: Wednesday	Off	
4: Thursday	Reverse Ball Crunches	Lower Rectus Abdominis
5: Friday	Ball Twists	Transversus Abdominis
6: Saturday	Ball Tuck Crunches	Upper/Lower Rectus Abdominis
7: Sunday	Off	

If you're a beginner or intermediate exerciser, here's your plan!

Week	For each exercise	Rest after each superset
1	3 sets, 10 reps	15 seconds
2	3 sets, 15 reps	20 seconds
3	3 sets, 20 reps	25 seconds
4	3 sets, 25 reps	30 seconds
5	3 sets, 30 reps	35 seconds

If you're an advanced exerciser, here's your plan!

Week	For each exercise	Rest after each superset
1	4 sets, 20 reps	10 seconds
2	4 sets, 25 reps	15 seconds
3	4 sets, 30 reps	20 seconds
4	4 sets, 35 reps	25 seconds
5	4 sets, 40 reps	30 seconds

You'll be doing more repetitions as the weeks go on. The rest time between sets also increases each week. The 5 core exercises—just like the exercises in Phases 2 and 3—will stay the same throughout the entire 5-week plan.

I wanted to lose pregnancy weight, plus get in shape for health reasons. But I was getting tired of working out and never seeing results. I was never a couch potato, so I became frustrated when I wasn't seeing any change in my body. 5-Factor changed that. I started to finally see muscle definition, and I love how little time it takes to complete a workout.

Holly Flom AGE: **37** WEIGHT LOST SO FAR: **29 lbs.**

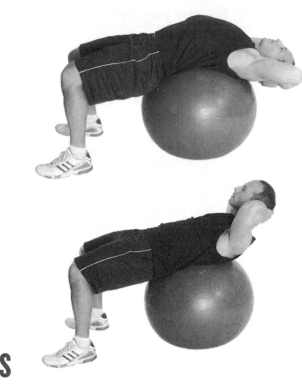

CORE EXERCISES
DAY I: MONDAY

BALL CRUNCHES

Sit on a stability ball with your feet flat on the floor. Place your hands along the sides of your head. Keeping your feet flat on the floor, slowly lean back until your head, shoulders, and back are all touching the ball. This is the starting position. Slowly curl your shoulders and upper back up off the ball. Lower yourself back down on the ball and repeat.

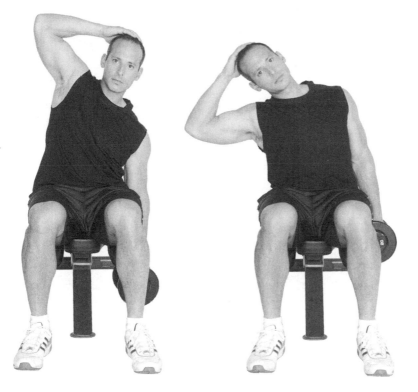

SEATED DUMBBELL SIDE BENDS

Sit on a chair or bench, holding a dumbbell in your left hand, palm facing in. Rest your right hand on the top of your head and let your left arm hang straight down along your side. Keeping your left arm straight, take a breath and bend at the waist to the right as far as you comfortably can. Return to the starting position, then bend at the waist to the left. Return to the starting position and repeat the exercise for the prescribed number of repetitions. Then switch positions, placing the weight in your right hand and your left hand on top of your head, and repeat the exercise.

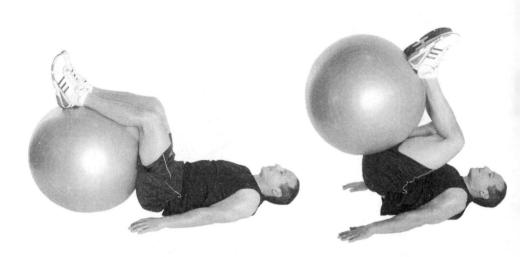

DAY 4: THURSDAY

REVERSE BALL CRUNCH

Lie flat on the floor faceup and with your knees bent. Place a stability ball behind your knees and draw your feet toward your butt to tuck the ball in place. Extend your arms straight down at your sides, with your palms pressed flat on the floor. This is the start position. Keeping the ball tucked underneath your legs, slowly curl your knees toward your chest. Pause, lower your legs back down until the ball touches the floor, and repeat.

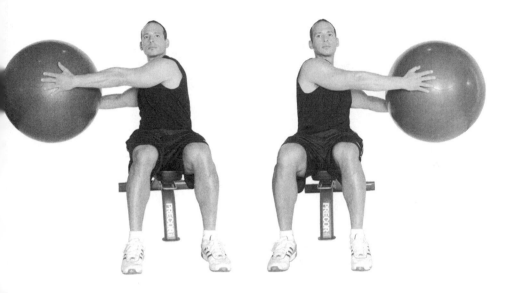

BALL TWISTS

Sit on a bench with your knees bent and your feet flat on the floor. Hold
a stability ball with both hands and extend your arms above your chest.
Keeping your arms straight, twist to the right. Bring the ball back to the front
so it's directly in front of you. Then repeat the move, this time twisting to the
left. Alternate right and left throughout the set.

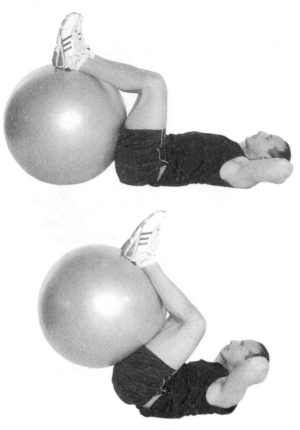

DAY 6: SATURDAY

BALL TUCK CRUNCH

Position yourself as if you were going to do a sit-up, but instead of keeping your feet on the floor, place them up on a stability ball. Your heels should press against the top of the ball. Keeping your arms bent behind your head, lift your hips and draw your knees toward your midsection—the ball should naturally roll toward your head. Hold, then extend your legs back until they're back in the starting position. Repeat.

PHASE 5: 5 MINUTES (OR LONGER) OF CARDIO WORK

For the last phase, go back to whatever activity you were doing in Phase 1. This time, it should feel easy to work at the same high intensity you achieved at the end of Phase 1. Start exercising, bring your pulse rate back up to your target BPM, and maintain that pace for 5 minutes. If you can go longer and have the time, go for it. The longer you can exercise, the more calories you'll burn overall. Personally, I would go for no more than 10 minutes total so I'd have enough energy for the next day's workout.

SUMMARY OF THE 5-FACTOR HOLLYWOOD WORKOUT
PHASE 1
Five minutes of cardio warm-up

PHASES 2 AND 3
Ten minutes of strength training

Day	Exercise	Core muscles involved
1: Monday	Incline Dumbbell Flys Ball Wall Squats	Chest Quadriceps
2: Tuesday	Reverse Incline Dumbbell Rows Dumbbell Deadlifts	Back Hamstrings
3: Wednesday	Off	
4: Thursday	Incline Dumbbell Bicep Curls Overhead Dumbbell Triceps Extensions	Biceps Triceps
5: Friday	Dumbbell Lateral Raises Step-Ups	Shoulders Quadriceps
6: Saturday	Bent-Over Dumbbell Rows Lying Ball Hamstring Curls	Back Hamstrings
7: Sunday	Off	

PHASE 4

Five minutes of core training

Day	Exercise	Core muscles involved
1: Monday	Ball Crunches	Upper Rectus Abdominis
2: Tuesday	Seated Dumbbell Side Bends	Lateral Obliques
3: Wednesday	Off	
4: Thursday	Reverse Ball Crunches	Lower Rectus Abdominis
5: Friday	Ball Twists	Transversus Abdominis
6: Saturday	Ball Tuck Crunches	Upper/Lower Rectus Abdominis
7: Sunday	Off	

PHASE 5

Five minutes of cardio work

THE 5-MONTH 5-FACTOR CHALLENGE

After you complete the 5-week 5-Factor program, you can repeat it for as long as you like. Its built-in variety makes it a constant challenge for your muscles, so they continue to reap the benefits with each and every cycle. If you're up for a new challenge, I've designed a 5-month plan that really keeps your body guessing—and the results coming!

Follow the same exercises in this chapter and do the required reps, sets, and rest intervals I've indicated in the chart on page 109. In the middle of the plan, you'll take a break from the strength training and core exercises by doing cardio for 25 minutes for all 5 workouts for a week. Are you up for my 5-Factor fitness challenge? Ready, set, go!

If you're an advanced exerciser, here's your plan!

Week	For each exercise	Rest after each superset
1	16 reps, 3 supersets	60 seconds
2	12 reps, 3 supersets	55 seconds
3	10 reps, 4 supersets	50 seconds
4	12 reps, 3 supersets	55 seconds
5	16 reps, 3 supersets	60 seconds
6	20 reps, 3 supersets	60 seconds
7	16 reps, 3 supersets	55 seconds
8	12 reps, 4 supersets	50 seconds
9	10 reps, 4 supersets	45 seconds
10	16 reps, 4 supersets	50 seconds
11	20 reps, 3 supersets	55 seconds
Cardio	25 minutes	
12	25 reps, 3 supersets	60 seconds
13	20 reps, 4 supersets	55 seconds
14	16 reps, 4 supersets	50 seconds
15	12 reps, 5 supersets	45 seconds
16	10 reps, 5 supersets	40 seconds
17	12 reps, 5 supersets	45 seconds
18	16 reps, 4 supersets	50 seconds
19	20 reps, 4 supersets	55 seconds
20	25 reps, 3 supersets	60 seconds

CHAPTER 10

5-Factor Recipes

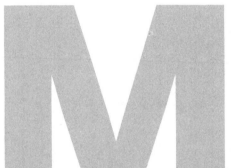

Most diet books tell you exactly what meals to eat and in what order. Who eats like that? I don't, and I know you don't either.

At the end of this book, I'll make suggestions for arranging my 120 5-Factor recipes into a weeklong plan. But whether you eat them in the recommended order is entirely up to you.

I want you to be creative. That's what makes the 5-Factor Diet so effective—and easy to stick to. Use these menus in whichever order keeps you coming back for more. When I work with Kanye West, for instance, he likes to eat the same thing for breakfast on most days: an egg white omelet with a little lean shredded beef and a bowl of berries. His favorite breakfast helps him stick to eating healthy.

Alicia Keys, on the other hand, loves to cook, and that gives her the ability to be more experimental. She enjoys variety in her diet and loves to try different 5-Factor menus.

If you want to eat the same breakfast every single morning, I have no problem with that. And if you prefer to mix things up every day, that's fine too. Each of the 120 recipes in this book is balanced nutritionally and specifically to meet the 5-Factor criteria. That way, even if you chose to eat the same five meals every day—or even the same meal five times a day!—you'd never be left nutrient-deficient.

I'm presenting you with 120 recipes—nearly a month's worth of meals—because variety is important to many dieters. These 120 fantastic recipes—just like the 100 recipes in *5-Factor Fitness*—not only are delicious but also are hands-down some of the easiest and most convenient recipes you'll ever try. I should know because I've had to make them on the fly for my clients at the strangest places and times.

FAST, FUN, AND DELICIOUS

When I'm on film sets with clients, I prepare their food quite often. I literally have minutes to make a meal when they unexpectedly take a break from filming. It was that kind of pressure that inspired my recipes.

Each had to be very simple to make.

Each had to use very few ingredients.

Each had to be delicious—I'm competing against catered food on sets, you know! (Halle Berry loves my 5-Factor fajitas, while Eva Mendes flips over my 5-Factor pizzas.)

And finally, each had to meet my 5-Factor criteria.

That's exactly what these recipes deliver. Not only do they fulfill the 5-Factor criteria, but they can be prepared—minus cook time—in just five minutes. You need only five—or fewer—core ingredients (plus seasonings and oils). I kept the number of steps in each recipe to five as well. If you want even more variety, I encourage you to check out the recipes in *5-Factor Fitness*.

It's easy to make 5-Factor meals and enjoy the benefits of the 5-Factor Diet. So let's get cooking!

No more excuses.

Meal 1. Breakfast

Asparagus Crepes with Toast

I bunch asparagus spears

1½ cups egg whites

⅔ cup nonfat milk

4 slices whole grain bread, toasted

Salt and cracked black pepper to taste

Cooking oil spray

1. Place the asparagus spears in a container with a little water. Microwave for 1½ minutes, then drain and set aside.

2. Whisk together the egg whites, milk, salt, and pepper.

3. Coat a nonstick skillet with cooking spray and heat the skillet. Pour half of the egg whites into the skillet. When the egg whites begin to set, turn them over. Cook for 30 seconds and then slide the crepe onto a cutting board. Place half of the asparagus spears in the center of the crepe and roll tightly. Repeat but reserve a couple of asparagus spears for garnish.

To Serve: Place the asparagus crepes on plates and serve with toast. Garnish with the reserved asparagus spears.

Servings: 2

Frittata Italiana

1. Whisk together the egg whites, cream cheese, salt, and pepper.

2. Spray a nonstick skillet with cooking spray and heat the skillet. Add the egg white mixture and cook until it begins to set. Immediately add the sun-dried tomatoes and basil leaves. Cover and cook about 2 minutes or until the eggs are completely set.

To Serve: Slide the frittata onto a cutting board and cut into four wedges. Serve two wedges and two slices of toast on each plate. Garnish with pepper and additional fresh basil.

Servings: 2

1½ cups egg whites

¼ cup nonfat cream cheese, softened

I cup finely chopped sun-dried tomatoes

4 leaves fresh basil, finely chopped

4 slices whole grain bread, toasted

Salt and cracked black pepper to taste

Cooking oil spray

Breakfast Burritos I

¾ cup egg whites

2 whole grain or whole wheat tortillas

2¼ cups canned black beans, drained

½ cup shredded nonfat mozzarella cheese

I cup salsa

I teaspoon ground cumin

I teaspoon garlic salt

Cracked black pepper to taste

Cooking oil spray

1. Preheat the oven or toaster oven to 350°F.

2. Whisk together the egg whites, cumin, garlic salt, and pepper. Coat a nonstick skillet with cooking spray and heat the skillet. Add the egg white mixture. Cook and stir over low heat until egg whites are cooked. Set aside.

3. Lay tortillas on a cutting board and sprinkle with black beans. Top with the egg whites and shredded cheese and roll tightly. Wrap the burritos in foil and bake for 2 minutes.

To Serve: Unwrap the burritos, cut in half, and serve with salsa.

Servings: 2

Breakfast Burritos II

1. Whisk together the ricotta cheese, egg whites, taco seasoning mix, onion powder, salt, and pepper. Stir in the tomatoes. Coat a nonstick skillet with cooking spray and heat the skillet. Add the egg mixture. Cook and stir until the egg whites are cooked. Set aside.

2. Heat the tortillas in the microwave for 20 seconds and place on a cutting board. Place the scrambled eggs and spinach in the center of each tortilla. Roll tightly.

To Serve: Cut the burritos in half and serve hot.

Servings: 2

I cup nonfat ricotta cheese

¼ cup egg whites

4 cups diced tomatoes

4 whole grain or whole wheat tortillas

8 cups spinach leaves

2 teaspoons taco seasoning mix

I teaspoon onion powder

Salt and cracked black pepper to taste

Cooking oil spray

Breakfast Burritos III

2 cups egg whites

2 large whole grain or whole wheat tortillas

1¼ cups refried beans

¼ cup shredded nonfat cheddar cheese

I cup salsa

Cooking oil spray

1. Coat a nonstick skillet with cooking spray and heat the skillet. Add the egg whites. Cook and stir for 1½ minutes. Set aside.

2. Heat the tortillas in the microwave for 15 seconds. Spread the tortillas with refried beans and spoon the egg whites over the beans. Sprinkle with cheese and roll the tortillas tightly.

To Serve: Cut the burritos in half and serve with salsa.

Servings: 2

Broccoli-Cheddar Omelet

1. Whisk together the egg whites, Mrs. Dash, salt, and pepper. Coat a nonstick skillet with cooking spray and heat the skillet. Add the broccoli florets and cook and stir until they are bright green. Add the egg whites and cook while gently pushing them to the center with a rubber spatula. When the egg mixture begins to set on the bottom, turn it over. Sprinkle with cheese and cover the pan. Cook for 30 seconds or until the cheese begins to melt.

To Serve: Slide the omelet onto a plate and fold in half. Cut in half and serve with toast.

Servings: 2

NOTE: You can use any green vegetable in your refrigerator in place of the broccoli.

I¼ cups egg whites

3 cups broccoli florets, coarsely chopped

¼ cup shredded nonfat cheddar cheese

4 slices whole grain bread, toasted

I teaspoon Mrs. Dash seasoning mix

Salt and cracked black pepper to taste

Cooking oil spray

Bell Pepper Pancakes
with Mozzarella and Crisp Bacon

1½ cups egg whites

2¾ cups diced bell peppers

1 tablespoon nonfat sour cream

¼ cup shredded nonfat mozzarella cheese

2 strips turkey bacon

Salt and cracked black pepper to taste

Cooking oil spray

1. Preheat broiler. Whisk together the egg whites, bell peppers, sour cream, salt, and pepper.

2. Coat a nonstick crepe pan with cooking spray and heat the pan. Ladle ¼ cup of the egg white mixture into the pan and cook until it is partially set. Turn it over and cook until almost set. Repeat with the remaining egg white mixture. Place the pancakes on a nonstick baking sheet and sprinkle with the mozzarella cheese. Broil until the cheese is melted and golden brown.

3. Microwave the turkey bacon for 3 minutes.

To Serve: Transfer the pancakes and turkey bacon to serving plates.

Servings: 2

The Cowboy Omelet

1. Microwave the sweet potatoes for 3 minutes each. Peel the potatoes and set aside.

2. Whisk together the egg whites, chili powder, garlic powder, salt, and pepper. Coat a nonstick skillet with cooking spray and heat the skillet. Add the mushrooms and cook until most of the liquid has evaporated. Add the egg white mixture and cook until it begins to set. Add the Canadian bacon and cheddar cheese. Cover and cook until the cheese is melted.

To Serve: Cut the sweet potatoes into cubes and gently toss with the cinnamon, salt, and pepper. Cut the omelet in half and serve with the sweet potatoes.

Servings: 2

2 medium sweet potatoes

I cup egg whites

5 cups sliced button mushrooms

I ounce Canadian bacon, cut into thin strips

I cup shredded nonfat cheddar cheese

I teaspoon chili powder

½ teaspoon garlic powder

Salt and cracked black pepper to taste

Cooking oil spray

I pinch ground cinnamon

Egg and Veggie Muffins

1⅛ cups egg whites

1¾ cups broccoli florets, coarsely chopped

¾ cup diced red and green bell pepper

½ cup shredded nonfat mozzarella cheese

4 slices whole grain bread, toasted

Salt and cracked black pepper to taste

Cooking oil spray

1. Preheat the oven to 350°F.

2. Whisk together the egg whites, salt, and pepper. Coat 12 muffin cups with cooking spray. Pour the eggs into the muffin cups, filling each cup halfway. Drop the broccoli and bell pepper into the egg whites, dividing them evenly. Bake for 10 minutes or until the egg begins to set. Remove from the oven and sprinkle cheese over the top of each muffin. Return to the oven and bake until the egg has set completely and the cheese is melted and golden.

To Serve: Slide a knife around the edge of each muffin and unmold onto a cutting board. Cut in half or leave whole. Place on plates and serve with toast.

Servings: 2

Open-Face Egg and Bacon Sandwiches

1. Microwave the turkey bacon strips for 3 minutes or until crisp. Set aside.

2. Whisk together the egg whites, salt, and pepper. Coat a nonstick skillet with cooking spray and heat the skillet. Add the egg white mixture. Cook and stir about 1½ minutes or until the egg whites are set.

To Serve: Spoon the egg whites on the toast. Top with cheese, turkey bacon, and diced tomatoes.

Servings: 2

NOTE: If you can't find nonfat cheddar cheese, you can substitute shredded part-skim mozzarella cheese.

2 strips turkey bacon

1¼ cups egg whites

4 slices whole grain bread, toasted

½ cup shredded nonfat cheddar cheese

1¼ cups diced, seeded plum tomatoes

Salt and cracked black pepper to taste

Cooking oil spray

Red Bell Pepper Frittata with Baked Yams

2 cups egg whites

1½ cups coarsely chopped roasted red peppers

I cup shredded nonfat mozzarella cheese

2 large yams

2 teaspoons onion powder

I teaspoon ground cumin

Salt and cracked black pepper to taste

Cooking oil spray

1. Whisk together the egg whites, onion powder, cumin, salt, and black pepper. Stir in the roasted peppers and shredded cheese. Coat a small glass baking dish with cooking spray. Pour the egg white mixture into the baking dish. Microwave for 4 minutes. Set aside. Microwave the yams for 3½ minutes each. Cut the yams in half and season with salt and pepper.

To Serve: Cut the frittata and serve with yams. Garnish with cracked black pepper.

Servings: 2

Salmon-Leek Frittata with Whole Grain Toast

1. Whisk together the egg whites, leeks, salt, and pepper. Coat a small glass baking dish with cooking spray. Pour the egg white mixture into the baking dish. Cover with plastic wrap three-fourths of the way. Microwave for 4 minutes. Cool for 3 minutes.

To Serve: Run a knife around the edge of the frittata and turn it over onto a cutting board. Spread the frittata with cream cheese and top with chopped salmon. Cut frittata in half and serve with toast. Garnish with parsley and additional pepper.

Servings: 2

1½ cups egg whites

I cup sliced leeks (white part only)

2 tablespoons nonfat cream cheese

2 ounces smoked salmon, chopped

4 slices whole grain bread, toasted

Salt and cracked black pepper

Cooking oil spray

2 teaspoons dried parsley

Scrambled Egg Casserole

I plum tomato, seeded and diced

I tablespoon thinly sliced scallion, white part only

¾ cup egg whites

½ cup shredded nonfat mozzarella cheese

4 slices whole grain bread, toasted

Cooking oil spray

Salt and cracked black pepper to taste

1. Coat a nonstick skillet with cooking spray and heat the skillet. Add the tomato and scallion and cook until the scallion is light golden. Whisk in the egg whites and half of the shredded cheese. Cook and stir until the egg white mixture is almost set. Season with salt and pepper.

To Serve: Spoon the scrambled eggs into a small casserole and sprinkle with the remaining cheese. Microwave until the cheese is melted. Serve with toast.

Servings: 2

Scrambled Eggs with Toast and Grapefruit

1. Coat a nonstick skillet with cooking spray and heat the skillet. Add the cubed chicken and egg whites. Season with salt and pepper and cook for 2 minutes. Add the cheese and cook until the cheese is melted.

To Serve: Spoon the scrambled eggs onto plates and serve with toast and grapefruit.

Servings: 2

¼ pound smoked chicken breast, cut into cubes

¼ cup egg whites

½ cup shredded nonfat cheddar cheese

4 slices whole grain bread, toasted

2 grapefruit, cut in half and seeded

Cooking oil spray

Salt and cracked black pepper to taste

Smoked Salmon Omelet with Cream Cheese and Whole Grain Toast

I cup egg whites

¼ cup nonfat cream cheese, softened

2 ounces smoked salmon

4 slices whole grain bread, toasted

1¾ cups orange sections

Salt and cracked black pepper to taste

Cooking oil spray

1. Whisk together the egg whites, cream cheese, salt, and pepper. Coat a nonstick skillet with cooking spray and heat the skillet. Pour the egg white mixture into the skillet. Gently push the egg whites toward the center as they cook. When they are almost set, place the smoked salmon on top. Cover the pan and cook for 30 seconds. Remove the lid and season with additional pepper.

To serve: Slide the omelet onto a cutting board and fold in half. Cut the omelet in half and serve with toast and orange segments.

Servings: 2

Smoked Turkey and Tomato Scrambled Eggs with Toast

1. Coat a nonstick skillet with cooking spray and heat the skillet. Add the egg whites and cook for 30 seconds. Sprinkle with chopped turkey, tomatoes, and shredded cheese. Cook and stir about 2 minutes or until the egg whites are completely set. Season with salt and pepper.

To Serve: Serve the scrambled eggs with toast.

Servings: 2

NOTE: For lunch, spoon the scrambled eggs on toast and eat it as an open-face sandwich.

I cup egg whites

3 ounces deli-style fat-free smoked turkey, chopped

1½ cups chopped plum tomatoes

½ cup shredded nonfat mozzarella cheese

4 slices whole grain bread, toasted

Cooking oil spray

Salt and cracked black pepper to taste

Sweet Potato Home Fries and Scrambled Eggs

2 large sweet potatoes

½ cup diced Spanish onion

I bell pepper, seeded and diced

I cup egg whites

I cup shredded nonfat cheddar cheese

Cooking oil spray

1½ teaspoons garlic powder

I teaspoon paprika

I teaspoon red pepper flakes

Salt and cracked black pepper to taste

1. Microwave the sweet potatoes for 3½ minutes each or until tender. Peel off the skins and dice the potatoes. Coat a nonstick skillet with cooking spray and heat the skillet. Add the onion and cook for 1 minute. Add the sweet potatoes, bell pepper, garlic powder, paprika, and red pepper flakes. Toss gently and set aside.

2. Coat a nonstick skillet with cooking spray and heat the skillet. Add the egg whites, cheese, salt, and cracked black pepper. Cook and stir until the egg whites are set.

To Serve: Spoon the scrambled eggs and home fries onto plates. Garnish with cracked black pepper.

Servings: 2

NOTE: If you can't find nonfat cheddar cheese, use shredded part-skim mozzarella.

Ham Steaks with Applesauce and Toast

1. Place the ham steaks in a hot nonstick skillet and cook for 1 minute on each side. In a bowl, toss together the apple pieces, cinnamon, and sugar substitute. Microwave for 2 minutes. Mash the cooked apples and the cottage cheese with a fork.

To Serve: Serve ham steaks with applesauce and toast.

Servings: 2

⅓ pound extra lean ham, cut into two serving-size pieces

2¾ cups peeled, cored, and cut-up Fuji apples

½ cup nonfat cottage cheese

2 slices whole grain bread, toasted

1 teaspoon ground cinnamon

¼ teaspoon sugar substitute

Bran Pancakes with Ricotta

½ cup bran flakes

½ cup egg whites

½ cup nonfat sour cream

1¾ cups nonfat ricotta cheese

1 tablespoon sugar substitute

1 pinch salt

Butter-flavor cooking oil spray

2 teaspoons ground cinnamon

1. Whisk together the bran flakes, egg whites, sour cream, sugar substitute, and salt. Coat a nonstick skillet with cooking spray and heat the skillet. Ladle a thin layer of batter into the skillet. Cook until the batter begins to set. Carefully turn the pancake and cook on the other side until the pancake is completely set and is a light golden color. Repeat with the remaining batter.

To Serve: Dust the pancakes with cinnamon and serve with ricotta.

Servings: 2

Oatmeal-Berry Pancakes

1. Beat together the egg whites, strawberries, rolled oats, and sugar substitute until smooth.

2. Coat a nonstick skillet with cooking spray and heat the skillet. Ladle ¼ cup of the batter into the skillet. Cook until the batter is set around the edges of the pan, then push it toward the center with a spatula. Cook until the batter begins to set in the center. Turn the pancake over or cover the pan. Cook for 1 minute. Repeat with remaining batter.

To Serve: Slide the pancakes onto plates and top with sour cream. Garnish with blueberries.

Servings: 2

1½ cups egg whites

1⅓ cups chopped strawberries

1 cup rolled oats

1 cup nonfat sour cream

1 cup blueberries

1¼ teaspoons sugar substitute

Butter-flavor cooking oil spray

French Toast with Ricotta

⅔ cup egg whites

⅔ cup nonfat milk

2 slices whole grain bread

⅛ cup nonfat ricotta cheese

I teaspoon sugar substitute

I pinch salt

Cooking oil spray

I teaspoon ground cinnamon

1. Whisk together the egg whites, milk, sugar substitute, and salt. Soak the bread in the egg white mixture. Drain the excess liquid.

2. Coat a nonstick skillet with cooking spay and heat the skillet. Cook the bread, one slice at a time, until each side is set and bread is light brown.

To Serve: Place the French toast on a plate and top with ricotta. Garnish with cinnamon.

Servings: 1

Fully Charged Fruit Salad

1. Peel and section three of the oranges and squeeze the juice from the fourth orange. Whisk the orange juice, protein powder, and ginger into the cottage cheese.

To Serve: Spoon the cottage cheese into bowls and top with orange sections, apple wedges, and strawberries. Serve chilled.

Servings: 2

4 oranges

I scoop protein powder (100% whey)

I cup nonfat cottage cheese

2 Granny Smith apples, cored and cut into wedges

2 cups quartered strawberries

I teaspoon ground ginger

Cream of Wheat and Protein

2¼ cups nonfat milk

¾ cup Cream of Wheat

1 scoop protein powder (100% whey)

1 teaspoon ground cinnamon

1. In a saucepan, combine the milk, Cream of Wheat, and protein powder and bring to a boil. Whisk until smooth and creamy.

To Serve: Ladle into bowls and garnish with cinnamon.

Servings: 2

NOTE: If you can't find 100% whey protein, use soy protein.

Kashi GoLean with Nonfat Milk

To Serve: Place 1 cup of cereal in each bowl and add the milk.

Servings: 2

NOTE: You can find Kashi GoLean cereal in the organic section of your local market.

2 cups Kashi GoLean cereal or other high-fiber whole grain cereal

2 cups nonfat milk

Meals 2 and 4. Snacks

Apple-Turkey Roll-Ups with Relish and Mustard

5 ounces deli-style turkey breast, sliced

3 Granny Smith apples, cored and thinly sliced

2 tablespoons pickle relish

1 tablespoon whole grain mustard

1. Place the turkey slices on a cutting board. Lay the apple slices on the turkey and spread with relish and mustard. Roll tightly and secure each with a toothpick.

To Serve: Make the roll-ups ahead, wrap in plastic wrap, and refrigerate.

Servings: 2

Belgian Endive Stuffed with Cheesy Artichoke Spread

1. In a food processor, pulse the artichoke hearts, cream cheese, mozzarella cheese, parsley, onion powder, salt, and pepper.

To Serve: Pull the leaves from the endive and arrange them on a serving platter. Spoon the artichoke spread into the leaves.

Servings: 2

2 cups canned artichoke hearts, drained

½ cup nonfat cream cheese, softened

2 tablespoons shredded nonfat mozzarella cheese

I whole Belgian endive

I teaspoon dried parsley

I teaspoon onion powder

Salt and cracked black pepper to taste

Bruschetta

¾ cup finely chopped sun-dried tomatoes

4 whole grain crackers

⅔ cup shredded nonfat mozzarella cheese

I teaspoon garlic powder

½ teaspoon onion powder

I teaspoon Italian seasoning

Cracked black pepper to taste

1. Preheat broiler to medium. Spoon the sun-dried tomatoes onto the crackers and top with the mozzarella cheese. Season with garlic powder and onion powder. Broil until the cheese is melted.

To Serve: Garnish with Italian seasoning and pepper.

Servings: 2

Cheese Course

To Serve: Arrange the pear wedges on a plate and spoon the ricotta over the pears. Garnish with cracked black pepper.

Servings: 2

2 pears, cored and cut into wedges

I cup nonfat ricotta cheese

Cracked black pepper

Chicken and Swiss Bites

I ounce deli-style fat-free chicken breast, thinly sliced

4 ounces nonfat Swiss cheese, cut into strips

4 multigrain crackers

I cup salsa

To Serve: Roll the chicken slices around the Swiss cheese and arrange on top of the crackers. Garnish with salsa.

Servings: 2

Chicken Salad with Apples

1. In a small saucepan, cook the chicken in water until the chicken is fully cooked. Drain, cool, and dice the chicken.

2. In a mixing bowl, combine the chicken, apple, celery, sour cream, onion salt, and celery seeds. Cover and chill.

To Serve: Spoon the chicken salad into small bowls.

Servings: 2

2¾ ounces skinless, boneless chicken breast

2 cups peeled, cored, and diced Granny Smith apple

1¾ cups finely diced celery

1 cup nonfat sour cream

½ teaspoon celery seeds

1 tablespoon onion salt

Crunchy Celery Sticks with Roasted-Garlic Hummus and Smoked Turkey

I garlic clove, peeled

I cup cooked garbanzo beans, drained and rinsed

3 tablespoons freshly squeezed lemon juice

I stalk celery, cut into thick sticks

3 ounces deli-style sliced fat-free turkey

½ teaspoon olive oil

Salt and cracked black pepper to taste

I teaspoon dried parsley

1. Preheat the oven or toaster oven to 350°F. Wrap the garlic clove in foil and roast for 10 minutes. For the hummus, in a food processor, combine the roasted garlic, garbanzo beans, lemon juice, and olive oil. Pulse until a smooth paste forms. Season with salt and pepper. (If the hummus is too thick, add a little water until it reaches the desired consistency.)

To Serve: Arrange the celery sticks and turkey slices on plates. Serve the hummus in a small bowl and garnish with dried parsley.

Servings: 2

Edamame and Tuna Sashimi with Ginger-Scallion Vinaigrette

1. Cook edamame in boiling water for 2 minutes. Drain edamame and set aside. For vinaigrette, whisk together the water, soy sauce, ginger, and scallion. Toss the shredded carrots and tuna slices with the vinaigrette.

To Serve: Place the warm edamame in the center of a plate and season with a little salt. Arrange the carrots and tuna slices around the edamame.

Servings: 2

NOTE: Combining warm edamame with chilled tuna makes a refreshing hot and cold snack.

⅓ cup edamame beans, removed from pods

3 teaspoons grated ginger

3 teaspoons slivered scallion

3 cups shredded carrots

2¼ ounces sushi-grade yellowfin tuna, thinly sliced

½ cup water

I tablespoon soy sauce

Salt to taste

Grilled Chicken Kabobs with Carrot-Ginger Vinaigrette

I¾ cups shredded carrots

I Granny Smith apple, shredded

½ cup rice wine vinegar

5 ounces skinless, boneless chicken breast, cut into bite-size pieces

I bell pepper, seeded and cut into squares

I teaspoon ground ginger

Salt and cracked black pepper to taste

Cooking oil spray

1. In a blender or food processor, combine the carrots, apple, rice wine vinegar, ginger, salt, and cracked black pepper. Pulse until smooth. Pour into a container and refrigerate. If the vinaigrette is too thick, add a little water.

2. Alternately thread chicken and bell pepper pieces onto skewers. Coat lightly with cooking spray and season with salt and cracked black pepper. On a hot nonstick grill pan, cook the chicken skewers for 10 minutes or until the chicken is fully cooked.

To Serve: Place the chicken kabobs on plates and drizzle with the vinaigrette. Serve warm.

Servings: 2

NOTE: If you double this snack, you'll have a great lunch.

Chicken Slices with Cheese and Crackers

To Serve: Arrange the crackers on a plate and serve with chicken, cheese, and fruit slices.

Servings: 2

6 whole grain crackers or any high-fiber, low-sugar crackers

2 ounces deli-style smoked chicken, thinly sliced

2 ounces nonfat cheddar cheese, thinly sliced

½ peach, cored and thinly sliced

½ pear, pitted and thinly sliced

Pear and Arugula Salad with Ricotta

1 strip turkey bacon

1½ cups arugula leaves

2 pears, cored and thinly sliced

¾ cup nonfat ricotta cheese, softened

1 lemon, cut in half

Salt and cracked black pepper to taste

1. Microwave the turkey bacon for 2 minutes or until crisp. Crumble the bacon.

To Serve: Arrange the arugula on plates and top with the pear slices and crumbled turkey bacon. Spoon the ricotta around the plates. Squeeze the juice from the lemon over the salad. Season with salt and pepper.

Servings: 2

Roasted Asparagus Spears with Turkey Slices

1. Preheat the toaster oven to 350°F.

2. Toss the asparagus spears with cooking spray, salt, and pepper. Roast in the toaster oven for 4 minutes.

To Serve: Lay the turkey slices on a cutting board. Sprinkle with the shredded carrots and place roasted asparagus spears in the middle. Roll the turkey tightly around the carrots and asparagus. Garnish with sliced onion.

Servings: 2

20 asparagus spears

6 ounces deli-style fat-free turkey, thinly sliced

2 cups shredded carrots

½ cup very thinly sliced red onion

Cooking oil spray

Salt and cracked black pepper to taste

Smoked Turkey and Fruit Salad

1½ cups quartered strawberries

1 cup orange sections

1 Granny Smith apple, cut into wedges

1 ounce smoked turkey, cut into cubes

½ cup nonfat cottage cheese

1. Gently toss together the strawberries, orange sections, apple wedges, and turkey cubes. Refrigerate until ready to serve.

To Serve: Spoon the cottage cheese into bowls and top with the fruit mixture.

Servings: 2

Salmon Sashimi with Plums

1. Whisk together the soy sauce, garlic, ginger, wasabi powder, and sugar substitute.

2. Arrange half of the plums on a plate. Arrange all of the salmon over the plums. Arrange the remaining plums over the salmon. Pour the soy mixture over the plums. Refrigerate.

To Serve: Garnish with scallion and sesame seeds.

Servings: 2

I clove garlic, mashed

12 ounces plums, pitted and thinly sliced

3 ounces fresh salmon, sliced paper-thin

I scallion, thinly sliced

¼ cup low-sodium soy sauce

I teaspoon ground ginger

½ teaspoon wasabi powder

½ teaspoon sugar substitute

2 teaspoons sesame seeds

Egg Salad with Toast Points

4 hard-boiled eggs, yolks removed

I hard-boiled egg

2 tablespoons nonfat mayonnaise

2 stalks celery, finely diced

2 slices whole grain bread, toasted

I teaspoon onion powder

I pinch celery seeds

Salt and cracked black pepper to taste

1. Chop the egg whites and whole egg and place in a mixing bowl. Stir in the mayonnaise, celery, onion powder, celery seeds, salt, and pepper. Mix well.

To Serve: Cut the toast into quarters and serve with egg salad.

Servings: 2

Egg and Celery Platter with Mustard-Balsamic Sauce

1. Quarter the egg whites and set aside. Whisk together the sour cream, balsamic vinegar, mustard, salt, and pepper.

To Serve: Arrange the egg whites and celery sticks on a plate. Drizzle with the sauce and garnish with pepper.

Servings: 2

3 hard-boiled eggs, yolks removed

1¾ cups nonfat sour cream

½ cup balsamic vinegar

3 teaspoons Dijon mustard

4 stalks celery, cut into small sticks

Salt and cracked black pepper to taste

Hard-Boiled Eggs Stuffed with Tuna Salad

½ cup canned water-pack tuna, drained

½ cup nonfat sour cream

¼ cup thinly sliced scallions

2 hard-boiled eggs, halved and yolks removed

3 cups shredded carrots

I teaspoon onion powder

I teaspoon garlic powder

Salt and cracked black pepper to taste

1. In a bowl, combine the tuna, sour cream, scallions, onion powder, garlic powder, salt, and pepper. Stir until the ingredients are combined. Stuff the egg whites with the tuna mixture.

To Serve: Make a shredded carrot nest on a plate and top with the stuffed eggs. Garnish with pepper.

Servings: 2

Spinach Frittata and Toast

1. Whisk together the egg whites, onion powder, garlic salt, and pepper. Coat a nonstick skillet with cooking spray and heat the skillet. Add the egg white mixture and cook until it begins to set. Add the spinach and cover the pan. Cook until the eggs begin to set on top. Sprinkle the cheese over the frittata and cook until cheese is melted.

To Serve: Cut frittata into wedges and serve hot or cold with toast.

Servings: 2

½ cup egg whites

4 cups spinach

2 tablespoons shredded part-skim-milk mozzarella cheese

4 slices whole wheat bread, toasted

I pinch onion powder

I pinch garlic salt

Cracked black pepper to taste

Olive oil cooking spray

Hot Dog Skewers with Cherry Tomatoes and Pickles

4 veggie hot dogs

3 cups halved button mushrooms

2 cups cherry tomatoes

I cup pickles cut into chunks

3 tablespoons Dijon mustard

1. Microwave the veggie hot dogs for 1½ minutes. Cut each hot dog into four pieces. Alternately thread hot dog pieces, mushrooms, tomatoes, and pickles on skewers.

To Serve: Serve warm or cold with Dijon mustard.

Servings: 2

Roast Beef with Carrot-Pear Slaw

1. Lightly toss together the shredded carrots, pear, and lime juice. Combine the sour cream and horseradish and gently stir into the carrot mixture.

To Serve: Season the roast beef with salt and pepper and serve with the coleslaw.

Servings: 2

1½ cups shredded carrots

I pear, cored and chopped

¼ cup nonfat sour cream

I tablespoon horseradish

4 ounces deli-style roast beef, thinly sliced

I teaspoon lime juice

Salt and cracked black pepper to taste

Spicy Jumbo Shrimp with Black Bean Dip

6 jumbo shrimp, peeled and deveined

1⅓ cups canned black beans, drained

¼ cup finely diced red onion

I lime

4 tablespoons whole cilantro leaves

I teaspoon red pepper flakes

Salt and cracked black pepper to taste

Cooking oil spray

1. Season the shrimp with half of the red pepper flakes, salt, and cracked black pepper. Coat a nonstick skillet with cooking spray and heat skillet. Add the shrimp and cook for 2 minutes or until the shrimp turn opaque.

2. Combine the black beans and red onion with the juice from one half of the lime, cilantro, remaining red pepper flakes, salt, and cracked black pepper.

To Serve: Place the black bean mixture in a bowl and serve with the shrimp. Slice the remaining lime half and garnish with the lime slices.

Servings: 2

Carrot Sticks with Onion Dip

1. Beat together the sour cream, cream cheese, and onion soup mix until very smooth.

To Serve: Arrange the carrot sticks on a plate and serve with the onion dip.

Servings: 2

¾ cup nonfat sour cream

½ cup nonfat cream cheese

1 tablespoon dry onion soup mix

12 ounces carrots, cut into sticks

Spinach Dip with Carrot Sticks

1¼ pounds spinach leaves

1 cup nonfat sour cream

¼ cup shredded nonfat mozzarella cheese

3 carrots, cut into 2-inch sticks

1 teaspoon onion powder

1 teaspoon garlic powder

Salt and cracked black pepper to taste

1. Combine the spinach, sour cream, mozzarella, onion powder, garlic powder, salt, and pepper in a plastic container. Microwave for 1½ minutes and stir.

To Serve: Serve the spinach dip with the carrot sticks.

Servings: 2

Smoked Salmon Mousse with Crackers

1. In a food processor, combine the smoked salmon, cream cheese, lemon juice, salt, and pepper. Pulse until smooth.

To Serve: Spoon the salmon mixture onto a plate and arrange the crackers around the plate. Garnish with dried dill and additional pepper.

Servings: 2

2 ounces smoked salmon

¼ cup nonfat cream cheese

6 tablespoons freshly squeezed lemon juice

6 multigrain crackers or any high-fiber, low-sugar crackers

Salt and cracked black pepper to taste

I teaspoon dried dill

White Bean Dip

½ cup nonfat cream cheese

⅓ cup drained white navy beans

I tablespoon freshly squeezed lemon juice

I stalk celery, cut into sticks

Salt and cracked black pepper to taste

1. In a food processor, combine cream cheese, navy beans, lemon juice, salt, and pepper. Pulse until a smooth paste forms.

To Serve: Arrange the celery sticks on a plate and serve with bean dip.

Servings: 2

Chips and Salsa

1. Preheat oven to 375°F. Put the tortilla triangles on a baking pan and bake until they are crisp. Set aside and cool.

To Serve: Place the tortillas in two shallow bowls. Dollop sour cream on the chips. Spoon the salsa over the sour cream. Sprinkle the cheddar cheese on top and garnish with scallion.

Servings: 2

3 large whole grain or whole wheat tortillas, cut into triangles

½ tablespoon nonfat sour cream

I cup salsa

½ cup shredded nonfat cheddar cheese

I scallion, thinly sliced

Pesto Crisps with Tomatoes and Cheese

¾ cup nonfat ricotta cheese

6 multigrain crackers (pesto or any Italian flavor)

8 small tomatoes, sliced

2 tablespoons basil leaves

Salt and cracked black pepper to taste

1. Spread a generous amount of ricotta on each cracker. Season the tomatoes with salt and arrange them on top of the crackers.

To Serve: Sprinkle the tomatoes with pepper and garnish with basil leaves.

Servings: 2

Sauteed Apples over Rice Cakes

1. Spray a nonstick skillet with cooking spray and heat the skillet. Add the apple wedges and cook until they begin to soften. Season apples with cinnamon.

To Serve: Place the rice cakes on plates and top with the cottage cheese. Arrange the apples over the cheese. Garnish with chopped turkey jerky.

Servings: 2

NOTE: The saltiness of the turkey jerky balances with the sweetness of the apples.

2 Granny Smith apples, peeled, cored, and cut into wedges

4 rice cakes

1 tablespoon low-fat cottage cheese

1½ ounces smoked turkey jerky, finely chopped

Cooking oil spray

1 pinch ground cinnamon

Pears with Peanut Butter Dip

⅓ cup nonfat cream cheese

2 teaspoons peanut butter

2 pears, cored and cut into wedges

1. Combine the cream cheese and peanut butter.

To Serve: Spoon the cream cheese mixture over the pear wedges.

Servings: 2

Cottage Cheese and Pears

1. Toss the pear wedges with the lemon juice. Combine the cottage cheese and the sugar substitute.

To Serve: Serve the pear wedges with the cottage cheese as a dip.

Servings: 2

2 pears, cored and cut into wedges

I teaspoon freshly squeezed lemon juice

I¼ cups nonfat cottage cheese

I ½ teaspoons sugar substitute

Fruit Skewers with Cottage Cheese

I pear, cored and cut into cubes

I teaspoon freshly squeezed lemon juice

20 strawberries, stems removed

I peach, pitted and cut into cubes

1⅛ cups nonfat cottage cheese

1. Lightly toss the pear cubes with the lemon juice.

2. Thread the pear cubes, strawberries, and peach cubes onto skewers. Chill until serving.

To Serve: Serve the fruit skewers with the cottage cheese.

Servings: 2

NOTE: You may also choose other 5-Factor-friendly fruits for this recipe.

Strawberry-Oatmeal Bars with Yogurt

1. Preheat the oven to 300°F. Combine the strawberries, rolled oats, egg whites, and 1 teaspoon of sugar substitute.

2. Coat a shallow baking dish with the cooking spray. Pour the strawberry mixture into the baking dish. Bake for 15 to 20 minutes. Set aside and cool.

3. Increase oven temperature to 425°F. Slice the cake into bars. Recoat the baking dish with cooking spray. Place the bars back in the baking dish. Bake for 5 minutes more or until crisp and golden. Cool.

To Serve: Stir the remaining sugar substitute into the yogurt. Serve the bars with yogurt for dipping.

Servings: 2

I cup sliced strawberries

½ cup rolled oats

½ cup egg whites

½ cup nonfat plain yogurt

2 teaspoons sugar substitute

Cooking oil spray

Toast with Berries and Cocoa Cottage Cheese

I cup fresh berries

2 slices whole grain bread, toasted

½ cup low-fat cottage cheese

I tablespoon unsweetened cocoa powder

2 teaspoons sugar substitute

1. Crush the berries with a fork and spoon them over the toast. Combine the cottage cheese, cocoa powder, and sugar substitute.

To Serve: Serve the toast with berries with the cottage cheese.

Servings: 2

Butterscotch and Apple Pudding

1. Place the apple in a container with 2 tablespoons water. Microwave for 2 minutes and set aside to cool. Whisk the pudding mix and the milk until smooth. Fold in the apple.

To Serve: Spoon ½ cup of ricotta cheese into each of two small glass bowls. Spoon the instant pudding on top.

Servings: 2

I Fuji apple, peeled, cored, and diced

I packet sugar-free, fat-free butterscotch instant pudding mix

1½ cups cold nonfat milk

I cup nonfat ricotta cheese, softened

Cheesecake

1½ tablespoons unflavored gelatin powder

½ cup nonfat cream cheese

½ cup nonfat sour cream

3 cups strawberries

¼ cup water

3 teaspoons sugar substitute

3 teaspoons vanilla extract

1. In a bowl, dissolve the gelatin powder in the water. Stir in the cream cheese, sour cream, sugar substitute, and vanilla extract. Pour the gelatin mixture into a glass baking dish and refrigerate until set.

To Serve: Spoon cheesecake onto plates and top with strawberries.

Servings: 2

Chocolate-Berry Parfaits

1. Whisk together the chocolate pudding mix and nonfat milk until smooth. In another bowl, whisk together the cottage cheese, yogurt, and sugar substitute.

To Serve: Spoon 1 tablespoon of pudding into each serving glass. Top with 1 tablespoon of the cottage cheese mixture and several raspberries. Repeat until all ingredients are used. Garnish with additional raspberries.

Servings: 2

I package fat-free, sugar-free chocolate-flavor pudding mix

I cup nonfat milk

¾ cup nonfat cottage cheese

½ cup nonfat plain yogurt

1¼ cups fresh raspberries

I teaspoon sugar substitute

Espresso Panna Cotta

I cup nonfat plain yogurt

I cup nonfat sour cream or quark

I shot espresso coffee, chilled

I tablespoon finely chopped bittersweet chocolate

3 teaspoons vanilla extract

2 teaspoons sugar substitute

1. Whisk together the yogurt, sour cream, coffee, chopped chocolate, vanilla extract, and sugar substitute until smooth. Pour into two small containers and chill until ready to serve.

To Serve: Serve chilled.

Servings: 2

NOTE: If you want to avoid caffeine, use decaf espresso. You can also try adding a fat-free, sugar-free coffee flavoring such as hazelnut or Irish cream.

Fresh Figs with Balsamic Cream Sauce

1. In a food processor, combine the cottage cheese, sour cream, balsamic vinegar, and sugar substitute. Process until smooth.

To Serve: Arrange the fig quarters on plates and pour the sauce over the figs. Garnish with pepper.

Servings: 2

I cup nonfat cottage cheese

2 tablespoons nonfat sour cream

½ tablespoon balsamic vinegar

6 figs, quartered

I teaspoon sugar substitute

Cracked black pepper to taste

Apple Wedges with Cinnamon Cream

I Granny Smith apple, cored and cut into wedges

I teaspoon freshly squeezed lemon juice

I cup nonfat sour cream

¾ cup nonfat cream cheese, softened

2 teaspoons ground cinnamon

2 teaspoons sugar substitute

1. Toss the apple wedges with the lemon juice. Whisk together the sour cream, cream cheese, cinnamon, and sugar substitute. Microwave for 30 seconds.

To Serve: Place the apple wedges on plates and top with the cinnamon cream.

Servings: 2

Sauteed Peaches with Cheese

1. Coat a nonstick skillet with cooking spray and heat the skillet. Place the peach wedges flat on the skillet and cook until they begin to soften. Turn each wedge over and cook other side.

To Serve: Spoon nonfat ricotta into small bowls and top with the peach wedges. Sprinkle with the sugar substitute and serve immediately.

Servings: 2

Note: If you do not have peaches, substitute apples or pears.

1⅜ pounds peaches, pitted and cut into wedges

I cup nonfat ricotta cheese

Cooking oil spray

2 teaspoons sugar substitute

Gelatin with Berries and Yogurt

1 package sugar-free raspberry-flavor gelatin

⅔ cup nonfat plain yogurt

3 cups quartered strawberries

2 cups raspberries

⅓ cup blueberries

1. Prepare the gelatin according to the package instructions. Pour the gelatin mixture into ice cream bowls and refrigerate until set.

To serve: Spoon yogurt on top of the gelatin and serve with strawberries, raspberries, and blueberries.

Servings: 2

Raspberry Gelatin with Cottage Cheese

1. Prepare the raspberry gelatin according to the package instructions. Pour the gelatin into pliable ice cube molds and place one raspberry in each cavity. Refrigerate until set.

To Serve: Unmold the gelatin cubes into a serving bowl. Gently toss the cottage cheese and remaining raspberries with the gelatin. Serve immediately.

Servings: 2

2 packages sugar-free raspberry-flavor gelatin

3½ cups fresh raspberries

1 cup nonfat cottage cheese

Lemon Yogurt with Kiwi

I cup nonfat plain yogurt

I cup nonfat sour cream

I tablespoon freshly squeezed lemon juice

2 sprigs fresh mint

2 kiwifruits, peeled and diced

I teaspoon sugar substitute

1. Whisk together the yogurt, sour cream, lemon juice, and sugar substitute. Chop one of the mint sprigs and combine with the kiwi.

To Serve: Place the yogurt mixture in small bowls and top with the kiwi. Garnish with the remaining mint leaves.

Servings: 2

Lemon Pie

1. In a bowl, dissolve the gelatin powder in the warm water. Stir in the cream cheese, sour cream, sugar substitute, and lemon extract until the mixture is smooth. Spoon into a pie plate and refrigerate until set.

To Serve: Spoon the lemon mixture into dishes and garnish with lemon zest.

Servings: 2

NOTE: Unflavored gelatin is sold in most markets in the pudding and gelatin section.

I tablespoon unflavored gelatin powder

½ cup nonfat cream cheese, softened

½ cup nonfat sour cream

¼ cup warm water

2 teaspoons sugar substitute

2 teaspoons lemon extract

2 teaspoons lemon zest

Chocolate-Mint Shakes

3½ cups quartered strawberries

2¼ cups nonfat milk

¾ scoop protein powder

I tablespoon unsweetened cocoa powder

I sprig fresh mint

1½ teaspoons sugar substitute

Crushed ice

1. Place the strawberries, milk, protein powder, cocoa powder, sugar substitute, and mint in a blender and pulse until smooth.

To Serve: Pour over crushed ice in tall glasses and serve immediately.

Servings: 2

Passion Fruit and Tangerine Shakes

1. Cut the passion fruits in half and scoop out the pulp and seeds. Place the passion fruit, tangerine sections, protein powder, and sugar substitute in a blender. Add the milk and pulse until smooth.

To Serve: Pour over crushed ice in tall glasses.

Servings: 2

NOTE: If you are unable to find fresh passion fruits, buy passion fruit pulp from the frozen section of your local market.

8 passion fruits

I cup tangerine sections

2 scoops protein powder (100% whey)

2¾ cups nonfat milk

2 teaspoons sugar substitute

Crushed ice

Tropical Berry Protein Shakes

2 passion fruits

I cup raspberries

¾ cup nonfat milk

I scoop protein powder (100% whey)

3 teaspoons sugar substitute

½ cup water

Crushed ice

1. Cut the passion fruits in half and spoon out the pulp. In a blender, combine the passion fruit pulp, raspberries, milk, protein powder, and sugar substitute. Add the water and pulse until smooth.

To Serve: Pour over crushed ice in tall glasses.

Servings: 2

NOTE: If you are not able to find passion fruits in your local market, use 3 tablespoons freshly squeezed orange juice.

Berry Protein Shakes

1. Combine the milk, raspberries, strawberries, protein powder, and vanilla extract in a blender. Blend until smooth.

To Serve: Pour over crushed ice in tall glasses and serve immediately.

Servings: 2

NOTE: Look for 100% whey protein powder in health food stores or in the fitness section of your local market. Or use soy protein powder.

2 cups nonfat milk

1½ cups raspberries

1 cup strawberries

½ scoop protein powder (100% whey)

1 teaspoon vanilla extract

Crushed ice

Meal 3. Lunch

4 cups canned artichoke hearts, drained

2 cups diced tomatoes

¾ cup cubed nonfat mozzarella cheese

2 ounces deli-style fat-free turkey, cubed

I cup fat-free balsamic vinaigrette

Cracked black pepper to taste

I teaspoon dried basil

1. In a bowl, toss together artichoke hearts, tomatoes, cheese, turkey cubes, balsamic vinaigrette, and pepper. Garnish with dried basil.

Servings: 2

Baked Chicken and Black Bean Quesadillas with Salsa

1. Combine the cumin, paprika, garlic powder, salt, and pepper. Season the chicken breast with the spice mixture. Coat a nonstick skillet with cooking spray and heat the skillet. Add the chicken and cook on medium heat until brown, turning once. Cover the pan and cook for 3 minutes more or until the chicken is fully cooked. Cool the chicken and slice into strips.

2. Preheat the toaster oven to 350°F. Place one tortilla on a cutting board. Arrange the sliced chicken on the tortilla and top with the black beans and mozzarella. Cover with the other tortilla and press down. Bake until the cheese is melted.

To Serve: Cut the quesadilla into quarters and serve with salsa.

Servings: 2

2 ounces skinless, boneless chicken breast

2 whole grain or whole wheat tortillas

I cup canned black beans, rinsed and drained

½ cup shredded nonfat mozzarella cheese

2 cups salsa

½ tablespoon ground cumin

½ tablespoon paprika

I teaspoon garlic powder

Salt and cracked black pepper to taste

Cooking oil spray

Baked Potato Skins with Sloppy Joe

2 large sweet potatoes

6 ounces ground chicken breast

½ cup tomato sauce

½ cup ketchup

2 cups diced tomatoes

2 tablespoons sloppy joe seasoning

I tablespoon garlic powder

I teaspoon onion powder

Salt and cracked black pepper to taste

2 teaspoons dried chives

1. Preheat the oven to 375°F. Wrap the sweet potatoes in foil and bake until tender. Remove potatoes from the oven and let cool for 10 minutes. Slice the sweet potatoes in half lengthwise and scoop out three-fourths of the pulp. The skins must remain intact. Place the potato skins in the oven and bake for another 8 minutes. Remove and set aside.

2. In a saucepan, combine the ground chicken, tomato sauce, ketchup, sloppy joe seasoning, garlic powder, onion powder, salt, and pepper. Cook over medium heat for 15 minutes. Add the tomatoes; cook 5 minutes more.

To Serve: Place the potato skins on plates and ladle the sloppy joe mixture over the potato skins. Garnish with dried chives.

Servings: 2

Black Bean Gumbo

1. In a medium saucepan, combine the water, chicken broth, and cubed chicken breast. Simmer for 15 minutes. Add the black beans, tomatoes, and Cajun seasoning and cook for 3 minutes.

To Serve: Ladle the soup into bowls.

Servings: 2

NOTE: If the soup seems too thick, add a little more chicken broth or water.

I cup fat-free chicken broth

2 ounces skinless, boneless chicken breast, cut into cubes

3 cups canned black beans, drained

2 cups diced tomatoes

3 cups water

2 tablespoons Cajun seasoning

Chicken and Rice Miso Soup

4 cups fat-free chicken broth

2 ounces skinless, boneless chicken breast

2 tablespoons miso paste or instant miso soup

1¾ cups cooked brown rice

I cup thinly sliced scallions

1. Combine the chicken broth, chicken breast, and miso paste or miso soup packet. Simmer about 20 minutes or until the chicken breast is no longer pink. Remove the chicken breast from the broth and dice it into small pieces.

2. Add the brown rice and the diced chicken to the soup and cook for 2 minutes.

To Serve: Ladle the soup into bowls and garnish with scallions.

Servings: 2

NOTE: Brown rice can be purchased precooked and heated 1 minute in the microwave. This alternative will save you time.

Chicken Fingers and French Fries

1. Preheat the oven or toaster oven to 375°F. Spread the sweet potato sticks on a sheet pan and lightly coat with cooking spray. Season with cinnamon, salt, and pepper. Bake for 25 minutes.

2. Dip the chicken strips into the egg whites, then drain off excess egg and coat with the ground bread. Coat a nonstick skillet with cooking spray and heat the skillet. Add the breaded chicken and cook until brown, turning once. Cook over medium-low heat for 5 minutes more.

3. Place the broccoli in a bowl with a little water and salt. Microwave for 2 minutes. Remove from the microwave and season with Mrs. Dash.

To Serve: Place the chicken fingers, sweet potato fries, and broccoli on plates.

Servings: 2

I large sweet potato, peeled and cut into sticks

5½ ounces skinless, boneless chicken breast, cut into strips

3 egg whites

4 slices stale whole grain bread, ground

4 cups broccoli florets

Cooking oil spray

I teaspoon ground cinnamon

Salt and cracked black pepper to taste

2 tablespoons Mrs. Dash Original Blend seasoning

Chinese Chicken Wraps with Peanut-Soy Sauce

5 ounces skinless, boneless chicken breast

I teaspoon unsalted peanut butter

¾ cup shredded carrots

4 large whole grain or whole wheat tortillas

¾ cup low-sodium soy sauce

I teaspoon ground ginger

I teaspoon ground coriander

I teaspoon dried chives

I teaspoon sugar substitute

1. Place the chicken breast in a saucepan, cover with water, and simmer until fully cooked. Remove from the heat and cut the chicken into small cubes.

2. Whisk together the soy sauce, ginger, coriander, chives, sugar substitute, and peanut butter. Place the chicken and shredded carrots in a Ziploc bag and add the soy sauce mixture. Seal and refrigerate for 15 minutes. Drain the chicken mixture.

To Serve: Place some of the chicken mixture on each tortilla. Roll tightly and cut into pieces. Serve warm or cold.

Servings: 2

Harley's Sweet Potato Melt

1. Microwave the sweet potatoes for 3½ minutes each or until tender. Cut in half and set aside.

2. Preheat the broiler or toaster oven broiler to medium. In a mixing bowl, combine the tuna, mayonnaise, Mrs. Dash, and lemon pepper.

To Serve: Place the tuna mixture on top of the sweet potato halves. Top with cheese and broil until the cheese has melted.

Servings: 2

Note: Tuna also comes with different flavorings. Try smoked tuna or tuna teriyaki by Starkist Creations.

2 large sweet potatoes

¾ cup water-pack canned tuna, drained

½ cup nonfat mayonnaise

½ cup shredded part-skim-milk mozzarella cheese

I teaspoon Mrs. Dash roasted garlic and onion seasoning

Lemon pepper to taste

Mediterranean-Style Chicken and Quinoa Salad

6 ounces skinless, boneless chicken breast

¾ cup quinoa

1⅓ cups diced, seeded plum tomatoes

I cup chopped fresh parsley

3 tablespoons freshly squeezed lemon juice

Salt and cracked black pepper to taste

1. Place the chicken breast and 2 cups of water in a small saucepan and cook for 8 minutes. Let the chicken cool and dice it. Set aside.

2. Put the quinoa and 1½ cups of water into a saucepan and simmer about 15 minutes or until the liquid is absorbed. Stir occasionally. Combine the chicken, quinoa, tomatoes, parsley, lemon juice, salt, and pepper; toss gently.

To Serve: Spoon the salad into shallow bowls.

Servings: 2

Mexican Chicken Salad with Spicy Salsa Dressing

1. Combine the fajita seasoning mix, cumin, salt, and pepper. Coat the chicken breast with the seasoning mixture. Microwave the chicken for 6 minutes. Remove from the microwave and set aside to cool slightly.

2. In a blender, combine the sour cream and salsa. Pulse until smooth. If the dressing is too thick, add a little water.

To Serve: Cut the chicken breast into ½-inch pieces and toss it with the lettuce, corn, and salsa dressing. Serve immediately.

Servings: 2

6 ounces skinless, boneless chicken breast

I cup nonfat sour cream

I cup salsa

I small head iceberg lettuce, coarsely chopped

1½ cups canned corn, drained

I teaspoon fajita seasoning mix

I pinch cumin

Salt and cracked black pepper to taste

Minestrone

4 cups chicken broth

2 cups canned stewed tomatoes

1⅓ cups thinly sliced button mushrooms

1⅓ cups cooked cannellini beans

1 cup diced smoked turkey breast

2 tablespoons dried basil

1 teaspoon sugar substitute

Salt and cracked black pepper to taste

1. In a saucepan combine the chicken broth, stewed tomatoes, sliced mushrooms, cannellini beans, turkey breast, basil, sugar substitute, salt, and pepper. Bring to a boil. Lower the temperature and simmer about 15 minutes or until the soup is reduced to half its volume.

To Serve: Ladle into soup bowls and serve immediately.

Servings: 2

Mixed Greens with Turkey and Cheese Quesadillas

1. Place the turkey slices on one side of each tortilla. Sprinkle with cheese and fold tortilla in half. Press tightly to secure the filling.

2. Coat a nonstick skillet with cooking spray and heat the skillet. Cook the tortillas for 1 minute on each side or until the cheese is melted. Slide the quesadillas onto a cutting board. Slice each into three or four triangles. Set aside.

To Serve: Toss the mixed greens with the salad dressing. Place the greens in the center of the plates. Arrange the quesadilla triangles around the salads.

Servings: 2

¼ pound deli-style sliced fat-free turkey

2 whole grain or whole wheat tortillas

½ cup shredded nonfat mozzarella cheese

3 cups mixed greens

I cup fat-free blue cheese salad dressing or other fat-free dressing

Cooking oil spray

Mushroom-Barley Risotto

3 cups sliced button mushrooms

I cup nonfat beef broth

½ cup pearl barley

3 ounces shrimp, peeled, deveined, and cut in half

I cup nonfat sour cream

4 cups water

I tablespoon dried sage

I tablespoon garlic powder

Salt and cracked black pepper to taste

1. In a large saucepan, combine the water, mushrooms, beef broth, and barley. Simmer for 15 minutes or until most of the liquid has been absorbed. Stir in the shrimp, sour cream, sage, garlic powder, salt, and pepper. Simmer for 2 minutes.

To Serve: Ladle the risotto into bowls and serve hot.

Servings: 2

Open-Face Turkey BLT

1. Microwave the turkey bacon for 3 minutes or until crisp. Crumble the bacon and set aside. Lay the romaine leaves flat on a plate. Layer with the sliced turkey, sliced tomatoes, and the turkey bacon. Season with salt and pepper and drizzle with red wine vinegar.

To Serve: Place the bun-less BLTs on plates and serve immediately.

Servings: 2

2 strips turkey bacon

I head romaine lettuce, leaves washed and patted dry

6 ounces deli-style fat-free turkey, thinly sliced

2 tomatoes, thinly sliced

I tablespoon red wine vinegar

Salt and cracked black pepper to taste

Pink Pizza

4 large whole grain or whole wheat tortillas

I cup tomato sauce

¾ cup nonfat ricotta cheese

I cup chopped sun-dried tomatoes

¾ cup shredded nonfat mozzarella cheese

1. Preheat the oven to 375°F. Place the tortillas on a baking sheet and bake for 2 minutes. Remove from the oven. Ladle half of the tomato sauce over the tortillas and spread with the ricotta cheese. Ladle on the remaining tomato sauce and sprinkle with sun-dried tomatoes and shredded mozzarella. Bake until the cheese is melted.

To Serve: Cut the pizzas into slices and serve immediately.

Servings: 2

Portobello and Turkey Stacks

1. Preheat the broiler to medium. Season the turkey breast with salt and pepper. Coat a nonstick skillet with cooking spray and heat the skillet. Add the turkey breast and cook until fully cooked, turning once. Slice thinly and set aside.

2. Lightly coat the mushroom caps with cooking spray and sprinkle with salt and pepper. Coat a nonstick skillet with cooking spray and heat the skillet. Add the mushrooms and cook until tender, turning once. Set aside.

To Assemble: Place the mushrooms on a sheet pan and top with the turkey. Place the tomato on top of the turkey and season with salt and pepper. Top with mozzarella. Broil until the cheese is melted.

To Serve: With a spatula, carefully slide the turkey stacks onto serving plates. Sprinkle with dried basil. Serve with crackers.

Servings: 2

4 ounces skinless, boneless turkey breast

4 portobello mushrooms, stems removed

1 tomato, thinly sliced

1 ounce fat-free mozzarella cheese, thinly sliced

10 whole grain or multigrain crackers

Salt and cracked black pepper to taste

Olive oil cooking spray

1 teaspoon dried basil

Salad Niçoise

12 ounces sweet potato

6 cups green beans, cooked

1½ cups water-pack tuna, drained

2 hard-boiled egg whites, chopped

½ cup fat-free Italian salad dressing

Salt and cracked black pepper to taste

1. Microwave the sweet potato for 3 minutes. Peel the potato and slice into ½-inch rounds. Set aside.

To Serve: Place the sweet potato rounds on serving plates. Arrange the green beans beside the sweet potato. Sprinkle the tuna and chopped egg whites around the green beans and sweet potatoes. Season with salt and pepper and drizzle with the salad dressing. Served chilled.

Servings: 2

Salmon Tartare with Arugula

1. In a bowl, combine the diced salmon, capers, juice from 1 of the lemons, onion and garlic salt, garlic powder, salt, and pepper.

To Serve: Arrange the arugula on a plate and season with salt and pepper. Sprinkle the salmon mixture over the arugula. Cut remaining lemon into wedges and garnish with wedges. Serve with crackers.

Servings: 2

6 ounces salmon fillets, finely diced

¼ cup capers, rinsed and chopped

2 lemons

I pound arugula

12 multigrain crackers

I tablespoon onion and garlic salt

I tablespoon garlic powder

Salt and cracked black pepper to taste

Greek-Style Shrimp and Spinach Salad

½ cup freshly squeezed lemon juice

1½ ounces feta cheese, crumbled

5 ounces shrimp, peeled and deveined

I pound spinach leaves

4 cups orange sections

2 teaspoons ground oregano

I teaspoon ground coriander

Salt and cracked black pepper to taste

1½ tablespoons Mrs. Dash seasoning

Cooking oil spray

1. Whisk together the lemon juice, feta cheese, oregano, coriander, salt, and pepper. Set aside. Season the shrimp with Mrs. Dash, salt, and pepper. Coat a nonstick skillet with cooking spray and heat the skillet until very hot. Add the shrimp and cook about 2 minutes or until shrimp are opaque.

To serve: Toss the feta mixture with the spinach and arrange on plates. Top with the shrimp and garnish with the orange sections.

Servings: 2

Smoked Salmon Pizza

1. Preheat the oven to 375°F. Place the tortillas on a baking sheet and bake for 4 minutes or until crisp.

To Serve: Spread the cream cheese on the tortillas and top with the tomato slices. Arrange the smoked salmon over the tomato and sprinkle with the red onion. Season with salt and pepper. Cut into wedges.

Servings: 2

4 whole grain or whole wheat tortillas

1 cup nonfat cream cheese, softened

2 tomatoes, thinly sliced

4 ounces thinly sliced smoked salmon

⅔ cup thinly sliced red onion

Salt and cracked black pepper to taste

Snapper Ceviche with Sweet Potato Rounds

2 medium sweet potatoes

10 ounces thinly sliced snapper fillet

1¼ cups freshly squeezed lemon juice

½ cup thinly sliced red onion

3 tablespoons chopped fresh cilantro

I teaspoon ground cumin

I pinch sugar substitute

Salt and cracked black pepper to taste

1. Microwave the sweet potatoes for 3 minutes each. Let the sweet potatoes cool, then peel. Slice into ½-inch rounds and set aside.

2. In a Ziploc bag, combine the snapper, lemon juice, red onion, cilantro, cumin, sugar substitute, salt, and pepper. Marinate the fish in the refrigerator for 15 to 20 minutes or until it is completely pickled. (The fish will be white and firm to the bite.)

To Serve: Arrange the sweet potato rounds on plates and spoon the snapper mixture on top.

Servings: 2

Green Bean Salad with Tuna and Grapefruit-Scallion Vinaigrette

1. In a saucepan, cook the green beans with a pinch of salt in boiling water for 2 minutes. Drain the beans and place them in an ice bath until cool. Drain again.

2. In a bowl, whisk together the rice vinegar, ginger, garlic powder, sesame seeds, salt, and pepper. Add two grapefruit sections to the vinaigrette and whisk until the segments fall apart. Place the green beans in a large bowl and toss with the tuna, scallions, and vinaigrette.

To Serve: Place salad on plates and garnish with the remaining grapefruit segments.

Servings: 2

2 pounds green beans, stems removed

I cup rice wine vinegar

2 small grapefruit, sectioned

8 ounces canned tuna, drained and flaked

½ bunch scallions, bias sliced

I teaspoon ground ginger

I teaspoon garlic powder

I teaspoon sesame seeds

Salt and cracked black pepper to taste

Stuffed Mushrooms and Greens

2 cups lump crabmeat

1¾ cups prepared bulgur

6 large button mushroom caps

5 cups mixed greens

½ cup fat-free red wine vinaigrette salad dressing

2 teaspoons paprika

I teaspoon dried mint

I teaspoon garlic powder

I teaspoon onion salt

Salt and cracked black pepper to taste

Cooking oil spray

1. Preheat the oven to 375°F. Combine crabmeat, bulgur, paprika, mint, garlic powder, onion salt, salt, and pepper. It should be just moist enough to hold together. Pack the crab and bulgur mixture into each mushroom cap. Lightly coat with cooking spray. Place in a baking pan and bake for 10 minutes.

To Serve: Season the greens with salt and pepper and toss with the red wine vinaigrette. Arrange the greens on plates and put the warm mushrooms on top. Serve immediately.

Servings: 2

NOTE: To prepare the bulgur, soak it in 3 cups water for 20 minutes, then drain.

Tuscan Tomato Soup

1. Preheat the oven to 400°F. Place tomatoes in a baking dish and lightly coat with cooking spray. Roast for 15 minutes. Remove from the oven and set aside.

2. In a saucepan, combine the chicken broth, garlic powder, onion powder, sugar substitute, salt, and pepper. Simmer the mixture until it is reduced to half its volume. In a blender, pulse the tomatoes until chunky. Stir the tomatoes into the chicken broth mixture. Whisk in the sour cream.

To Serve: Ladle the soup into bowls and garnish with dried basil.

Servings: 2

I cup canned stewed tomatoes

4 cups chicken broth

3 cups nonfat sour cream

Cooking oil spray

I tablespoon garlic powder

I tablespoon onion powder

I teaspoon sugar substitute

Salt and cracked black pepper to taste

I tablespoon dried basil

Meal 5. Dinner

2 small eggplants, thinly sliced lengthwise

I cup tomato sauce

I pound tomatoes, thinly sliced

I cup nonfat ricotta cheese, softened

¾ cup shredded nonfat mozzarella cheese

Salt and cracked black pepper to taste

Cooking oil spray

2 tablespoons dried basil

2 tablespoons Italian seasoning

1. Preheat the oven to 400°F. Season the eggplant slices with salt and pepper and roast for 15 minutes.

2. Coat a glass baking dish with cooking spray and cover the bottom with eggplant slices. Ladle some of the tomato sauce over the eggplant and top with some of the tomato slices. Sprinkle the tomato slices with basil, Italian seasoning, salt, and pepper. Spread ricotta over the tomatoes. Sprinkle with shredded mozzarella. Repeat the layers, ending with mozzarella.

3. Bake for 20 minutes. Increase the heat to broil until the cheese turns golden.

To Serve: Cut the lasagna into slices and garnish with additional Italian seasoning.

Servings: 2

Argentine-Style Steak Salad with Watercress and Mustard-Cilantro Vinaigrette

1. In a mixing bowl, whisk together the vinegar, Dijon mustard, cilantro, salt, and pepper. Set aside.

2. Season the bison steak with cumin, coriander, salt, and pepper. Coat a nonstick skillet with cooking spray and heat the skillet. Add the steak and sear on each side to desired doneness, turning once. Remove the steak from the skillet and let stand for 1 minute. Slice the steak.

To Serve: Toss the watercress with the vinaigrette and place it on plates. Top with steak slices and garnish with radish slices.

Servings: 2

NOTE: Bison is a very lean meat, and has the best flavor and texture when cooked to medium-rare.

¼ cup white wine vinegar

1½ teaspoons Dijon mustard

6 ounces bison steak

4 bunches watercress, washed and patted dry

5 radishes, thinly sliced

2 tablespoons dried cilantro

Salt and cracked black pepper to taste

1 teaspoon ground cumin

1 teaspoon ground coriander

Cooking oil spray

Chicken Chow Mein

6 ounces skinless, boneless chicken breast, cut into strips

5 cups thinly sliced carrots

3 cups snow peas, stems removed

2 cups bean sprouts

Cooking oil spray

I tablespoon sesame seeds

I tablespoon garlic powder

½ cup low-sodium soy sauce

1. Coat a wok with cooking spray and heat the wok. Add the chicken strips and stir-fry for 2 minutes. Add the carrots, snow peas, bean sprouts, sesame seeds, and garlic powder. Stir-fry for 1 minute. Add the soy sauce and cook for 1 minute.

To Serve: Ladle into shallow bowls and garnish with a few additional sesame seeds.

Servings: 2

Chicken Ropa Vieja

1. In a saucepan, bring salted water to a boil. Add the chicken and cook over medium heat for 10 to 15 minutes. Drain the cooked chicken and cool. Shred the chicken.

2. In a saucepan, combine the tomato sauce, bell pepper slices, cumin, sugar substitute, bay leaf, salt, and cracked black pepper. Add the shredded chicken and cook for 5 minutes. Microwave the corn for 2 minutes. Season with salt and cracked black pepper. Discard bay leaf.

To Serve: Spoon the chicken mixture into bowls and top with corn. Garnish with fresh cilantro.

Servings: 2

7½ ounces skinless, boneless chicken breast

12 ounces tomato sauce

1 red bell pepper, seeded and thinly sliced

2½ cups canned corn, drained

2 tablespoons cilantro leaves

1 teaspoon ground cumin

1 teaspoon sugar substitute

1 bay leaf

Salt and cracked black pepper to taste

Chiles Rellenos with Brown Rice

2 large poblano peppers

6 ounces ground turkey breast

½ cup canned black beans, rinsed and drained

3 tablespoons tomato paste

I½ cups cooked brown rice

Cooking oil spray

I tablespoon ground cumin

I pinch sugar substitute

Salt and cracked black pepper to taste

1. Preheat the oven to 400°F. Lightly coat the poblanos with cooking spray. Place them on a baking sheet and roast for 20 minutes or until the skins begin to char. Remove the peppers from the heat. Immediately place them in a bowl and cover with plastic wrap to cool.

2. Carefully peel the poblanos and slit each one through one side. Remove the seeds with a paring knife and rinse the peppers under cold water to wash out any remaining seeds. Leave the peppers as intact as possible. Set the peppers aside.

3. Coat a nonstick skillet with cooking spray and heat skillet. Add the ground turkey and cook until no longer pink. Add the black beans, tomato paste, cumin, sugar substitute, salt, and cracked black pepper. Stir until well mixed. Spoon the turkey filling into the peppers.

To Serve: Spoon the cooked rice onto plates and top with the chiles. Garnish with fresh cilantro leaves, if desired.

Servings: 2

Country-Style Ham Steaks with Yams and Corn on the Cob

1. Coat a nonstick skillet with cooking spray and heat the skillet. Add the ham steaks and sear on each side until golden brown. Microwave the yams for about 3½ minutes each. Peel and slice them into rounds and season with salt and pepper. Cook the corn in boiling water for 3 minutes.

To Serve: Place the ham steaks on plates and serve with sliced yams and corn on the cob.

Servings: 2

9 ounces ham steaks

2 large yams

3 ears corn on the cob, husked and cut in half

Cooking oil spray

Salt and cracked black pepper to taste

Cream of Broccoli Soup with Sauteed Shrimp

2⅛ cups chicken broth

8 ounces broccoli florets

2¼ cups chopped carrots

¾ cup leeks, white part only, coarsely chopped

8 ounces shrimp, peeled, deveined, and cut into pieces

I tablespoon garlic powder

Salt and cracked black pepper to taste

Cooking oil spray

1. In a large saucepan, bring the chicken broth to a boil and add the broccoli, carrots, leeks, garlic powder, salt, and pepper. Cook for 3 minutes or until the broccoli is bright green and tender to the fork. Remove from the heat and let cool slightly.

2. Ladle a portion of the broccoli mixture into a blender and pulse until it reaches a creamy consistency. Pour the blended soup into a large saucepan. Repeat until all the broccoli mixture is blended. Reheat the soup.

3. Coat a nonstick skillet with cooking spray and heat the skillet. Add the shrimp and season with salt and pepper. Cook about 2 minutes.

To Serve: Ladle the soup into bowls and garnish with shrimp.

Servings: 2

Creamy Lemon-Ginger Halibut with Corn on the Cob

1. Zest one lemon and squeeze out the juice. Whisk together the lemon zest, lemon juice, yogurt, coriander, ginger, salt, and pepper. Place the halibut fillets in a Ziploc bag and pour three-fourths of the yogurt mixture over the fish. Marinate for 5 minutes.

2. Meanwhile, place the corn in a plastic container with water. Microwave for 5 minutes. Season with salt and pepper and set aside.

3. Remove the fish from the marinade and place in a plastic container. Cover and microwave for 6 minutes or until fish flakes when tested with a fork.

To Serve: Place the fish and corn on plates. Spoon a little of the remaining yogurt mixture over the fish. Cut the remaining lemon into wedges and serve with fish.

Servings: 2

2 lemons

¾ cup nonfat plain yogurt

8 ounces boneless halibut fillet, cut into two portions

2 ears corn on the cob, husks removed

1 teaspoon ground coriander

1½ teaspoons ground ginger

Salt and cracked black pepper to taste

Crispy Chicken Tostadas

6 ounces skinless, boneless chicken breast

1½ cups thinly sliced Spanish onion

2 tablespoons freshly squeezed lime juice

4 medium whole grain or whole wheat tortillas

2 tablespoons nonfat sour cream

Salt and cracked black pepper to taste

I teaspoon olive oil

4 teaspoons dried cilantro

I teaspoon ground cumin

1. Place chicken in large saucepan and add water to cover, salt, and pepper. Cook over medium heat for 25 minutes or until the chicken is fully cooked. Remove the chicken, cool, and shred.

2. Heat the olive oil in a nonstick skillet. Add the onion and cook for 1 minute. Add the shredded chicken and stir constantly until it crisps. When most of the liquid has evaporated, drizzle the lime juice over the chicken and season with cilantro, cumin, salt, and pepper. Set aside. Bake the tortillas in a 350° oven until they are crisp and light golden.

To Serve: Place the tortillas on plates. Top with the chicken and sour cream.

Servings: 2

Bison Steak with Cauliflower-Carrot Mash and Brown Rice

1. In a medium saucepan, cook the carrots in lightly salted boiling water for 2 minutes. Add the cauliflower and cook for 3 minutes or until the cauliflower is tender. Drain the vegetables and place in a food processor. Pulse the vegetables with the sour cream, onion powder, salt, and pepper. Transfer to a bowl with lid and set aside.

2. Divide the steak into two portions. Season the steaks with steak seasoning, salt, and pepper. Coat a nonstick skillet with cooking spray and heat the skillet until very hot. Add the steaks and sear on both sides. Then reduce heat to medium-high and cook until they reach the desired doneness (bison is best served medium-rare). Remove from the heat and let the steaks stand for 1 minute.

To Serve: Place the cauliflower-carrot mash in the center of the plates. Slice the bison steaks and arrange the slices over the mash. Serve with brown rice.

Servings: 2

2¼ cups chopped carrots

3½ cups cauliflower florets

2 tablespoons nonfat sour cream

6½ ounces bison steak

1¼ cups cooked brown rice

1 tablespoon onion powder

Salt and cracked black pepper to taste

2 tablespoons Montreal steak seasoning

Cooking oil spray

Indian-Style Chicken with Curried Yogurt Sauce and Brown Rice

½ cup nonfat plain yogurt

I teaspoon curry powder

8 ounces skinless, boneless chicken breast, butterflied and thinly pounded

2 cups cooked brown rice

2½ cups thinly sliced, peeled cucumber

½ teaspoon ground coriander

⅛ teaspoon ground paprika

Salt and cracked black pepper to taste

Cooking oil spray

1. Combine the yogurt, curry powder, coriander, paprika, salt, and pepper. Pour three-fourths of the mixture into a Ziploc bag. Add the chicken, seal, and refrigerate for 20 minutes. Drain the chicken and discard the marinade. Coat a nonstick skillet with cooking spray and heat the skillet. Add the chicken and sear on each side until golden brown. Cover the pan and reduce the heat to medium. Cook for 1 minute more and remove from the heat.

To Serve: Place the chicken and brown rice on plates. Top the chicken with the remaining yogurt sauce and the sliced cucumbers.

Servings: 2

Lobster and Peas with Tomato-Basil Sauce and Barley

1. In a soup pot, combine the tomato sauce, barley, lobster, basil, seafood seasoning mix, sugar substitute, salt, and pepper. Cook and stir for 4 minutes. Taste and adjust the seasonings. Add the peas and cook for 1 to 2 minutes.

To Serve: Ladle into shallow bowls and garnish with additional fresh basil leaves.

Servings: 2

NOTE: For a less expensive dish, you can prepare this recipe with shrimp or chicken breast.

1½ cups tomato sauce

1¼ cups cooked barley

1¼ cups uncooked lobster, coarsely chopped

½ bunch fresh basil, chopped

1½ cups frozen green peas

1 teaspoon seafood seasoning mix

1 teaspoon sugar substitute

Salt and cracked black pepper to taste

Salmon with Cucumber-Dill Salad

9 ounces salmon steak

2 large sweet potatoes

½ cup nonfat sour cream

2 tablespoons chopped fresh dill

I cup thinly sliced, peeled cucumber

½ tablespoon lemon pepper

I teaspoon paprika

Salt and cracked black pepper to taste

Cooking oil spray

1. Cut the salmon steak into two portions and season with lemon pepper, paprika, and salt. Coat a nonstick skillet with cooking spray and heat the skillet. Place the salmon steaks in the skillet, skin sides up. Sear for 1 minute, then turn and cook until the salmon flakes when tested with a fork.

2. Microwave the sweet potatoes for 3½ minutes each or until tender. Peel and slice into thick rounds. Season with salt and pepper and set aside.

3. Meanwhile, whisk together the sour cream, dill, salt, and pepper. Stir in the cucumber slices.

To Serve: Spoon the cucumber mixture over the salmon. Serve with sweet potato rounds.

Servings: 2

Scallop Ratatouille

1. In a soup pot, combine the tomatoes, zucchini, eggplant, mushrooms, water, basil, oregano, sugar substitute, salt, and pepper. Cover and cook over medium heat for 5 minutes. Add the scallops and cook for 2½ minutes more.

To Serve: Ladle the soup into bowls and garnish with additional dried basil.

Servings: 2

3 cups canned crushed tomatoes

3 cups cubed zucchini

3 cups cubed eggplant

3 cups quartered button mushrooms

½ pound small scallops

1 ½ cups water

3 tablespoons dried basil

2 tablespoons dried oregano

1 pinch sugar substitute

Salt and cracked black pepper to taste

Seared Halibut with Creamed Spinach and Brown Rice

5 ounces halibut fillets

I pound spinach leaves

½ cup nonfat cream cheese

¼ cup nonfat sour cream

1⅔ cups cooked brown rice

I teaspoon lemon pepper

Salt and cracked black pepper to taste

Cooking oil spray

I tablespoon onion powder

2 teaspoons garlic powder

1. Season the halibut fillets with lemon pepper and salt. Coat a nonstick skillet with cooking spray and heat the skillet. Add the halibut and sear on each side. Then cover the pan and cook until the fish flakes when tested with a fork. Set aside.

2. Cook the spinach in a nonstick pan over medium heat until wilted. Transfer the spinach to a strainer and press out as much liquid as possible.

3. Return the spinach to the pan. Add the cream cheese, sour cream, onion powder, garlic powder, salt, and cracked black pepper. Cook and stir over medium heat until hot.

4. Microwave the brown rice for 1 minute.

To Serve: Place the brown rice on the center of each plate. Top with halibut and spoon the creamed spinach over the halibut.

Servings: 2

Seared Scallops with Orange Sauce and Broccoli-Cauliflower Saute

1. Coat a nonstick skillet with cooking spray and heat the skillet. Add the scallops and season with the curry powder, salt, and pepper. Cook until scallops are golden brown. Add the broccoli, cauliflower, and orange juice. Cook until the broccoli is bright green and tender to the fork.

To serve: Spoon the scallops and vegetables into shallow bowls. Drizzle with the orange sauce.

Servings: 2

10 ounces large scallops

I pound broccoli florets

I pound cauliflower florets

I cup freshly squeezed orange juice

Cooking oil spray

I teaspoon curry powder

Salt and cracked black pepper to taste

Shrimp and Tofu Soup

1½ cups cooked brown rice

4 ounces shrimp, peeled, deveined,
and cut in half

4 ounces firm tofu cut into I-inch cubes

3 tablespoons miso paste or instant
miso soup

4 cups water

I cup low-sodium soy sauce

1. In a large saucepan, combine the water, rice, soy sauce, shrimp, tofu, and miso. Simmer for 2 minutes or until the shrimp are opaque.

To Serve: Ladle into soup bowls.

Servings: 2

Shrimp and Rice Stir-Fry

1. Remove the tails from the shrimp and cut the shrimp into bite-size pieces.

2. Coat a nonstick skillet with cooking spray and heat the skillet. Add the shrimp and cook for 2 minutes. Remove from the heat and set the shrimp aside.

3. Coat the skillet with cooking spray and heat the skillet. Add the rice and garlic powder and cook for 1 minute, stirring constantly. Add the broccoli and cook until it is bright green. Add the shrimp, scallions, soy sauce, and sesame seeds. Cook for 1 minute longer.

To Serve: Spoon the stir-fried mixture onto plates.

Servings: 2

I pound shrimp, peeled and deveined

1½ cups cooked brown rice

2 cups broccoli florets

¼ cup slivered scallions

Cooking oil spray

½ tablespoon garlic powder

¼ cup low-sodium soy sauce

2 teaspoons sesame seeds

Southern-Style Baked Chicken with Black-Eyed Peas and Collard Greens

6 ounces skinless, boneless chicken breast

5 bunches collard greens, cut into strips

2 cloves garlic, minced

¼ cup balsamic vinegar

2¾ cups canned black-eyed peas, drained and rinsed

1 tablespoon Lawry's Seasoned Salt

Cooking oil spray

¼ cup water

1 teaspoon sugar substitute

Salt and cracked black pepper to taste

1. Preheat the oven to 375°F.

2. Sprinkle the chicken with seasoned salt. Coat a nonstick skillet with cooking spray and heat the skillet. Sear the chicken on both sides until golden and crisp around the edges. Put the chicken in a baking dish and bake for 10 minutes.

3. Coat a large nonstick skillet with cooking spray and heat the skillet. Add the collard greens and garlic and cook for 4 minutes or until the greens are bright green. Add the vinegar and water. Cook until most of the liquid has evaporated. Add the sugar substitute, salt, and pepper and set the greens aside.

4. Place the black-eyed peas in a bowl and season with salt and pepper. Microwave for 1 minute.

To Serve: Transfer the hot chicken breasts to a cutting board and cut into ½-inch slices. Place the collard greens on the plates and arrange the chicken slices on top. Ladle the black-eyed peas over the chicken.

Servings: 2

Soy-Poached Chicken with Vegetables and Brown Rice

1. In a saucepan, combine the chicken, water, and soy sauce. Simmer for 8 minutes or until chicken is no longer pink. Drain the chicken and set aside.

2. Meanwhile, remove edamame beans from the pods and cook in boiling water for 2 minutes. Place the carrots, ginger, and garlic powder in a container and microwave for 2 minutes. Drain the edamame beans and stir into the carrot mixture. Season with a little salt.

To Serve: Place the chicken on plates and spoon the cooked brown rice on top. Garnish with the vegetable mixture.

Servings: 2

8 ounces skinless, boneless chicken breast, pounded thin

I cup edamame beans

2 cups thinly sliced carrots

I¼ cups cooked brown rice

2 cups water

I cup low-sodium soy sauce

I teaspoon ground ginger

I teaspoon garlic powder

Salt to taste

Spaghetti and Meatballs

2 small spaghetti squash, cut in half
and seeded

I cup canned crushed tomatoes

6 ounces ground turkey breast

I egg white

4 slices whole grain bread, toasted and
ground into crumbs

Cooking oil spray

Salt and cracked black pepper to taste

I bay leaf

I tablespoon sugar substitute

2 teaspoons onion powder

2 teaspoons garlic powder

I teaspoon tomato paste

Chopped fresh parsley (optional)

1. Preheat the oven to 400°F. Lightly coat the squash with cooking spray and season with salt and pepper. Bake for 30 minutes or until tender. (Or microwave each squash half for 6 minutes).

3. In a saucepan, combine the tomatoes, bay leaf, sugar substitute, 1 teaspoon of the onion powder, 1 teaspoon of the garlic powder, salt, and pepper. Bring to a simmer. In a mixing bowl, combine the ground turkey, egg white, bread crumbs, tomato paste, remaining onion powder, remaining garlic powder, salt, and pepper. Mix well. Roll 1½-inch meatballs between the palms of your hands. Drop the meatballs into the tomato sauce and cook for 15 minutes.

To Serve: Shred the spaghetti squash with forks and place on plates. Ladle meatballs and tomato sauce over the squash. Sprinkle with chopped parsley, if desired.

Servings: 2

Turkey Fajitas

1. Coat a nonstick skillet with cooking spray and heat the skillet. Add the turkey strips and cook for 2 minutes. Add the onion and cook 1 minute longer. Add the bell pepper, fajita seasoning mix, garlic powder, chili powder, salt, and cracked black pepper. Stir well to mix and cook for 1 minute.

To Serve: Heat the tortillas in the microwave for 15 seconds. Spoon the turkey mixture onto the tortillas and garnish with sour cream.

Servings: 2

6 ounces skinless, boneless turkey breast, cut into strips

I cup sliced Spanish onion

I bell pepper, seeded and cut into strips

2 large whole grain or whole wheat tortillas

½ cup nonfat sour cream

Cooking oil spray

2 tablespoons fajita seasoning mix

I tablespoon garlic powder

2 teaspoons chili powder

Salt and cracked black pepper to taste

Warm White Bean, Beet, and Turkey Salad

8 ounces turkey breast cutlet, cut into
1-inch pieces

1²⁄₃ cups canned white beans, rinsed and
drained

4 ounces veggie pepperoni, chopped

¼ cup white wine vinegar

6 ounces canned beets, drained and sliced

Cooking oil spray

1 teaspoon dried oregano

1 teaspoon dried basil

Salt and cracked black pepper to taste

1. Spray a nonstick skillet with cooking spray and heat the skillet. Add the turkey pieces and sear on both sides. Cook about 2 minutes or until they are golden brown.

2. In a mixing bowl, combine the turkey, white beans, veggie pepperoni, vinegar, oregano, basil, salt, and pepper. Toss gently.

To Serve: Arrange the beet slices on plates and spoon the turkey mixture over the beets.

Servings: 2

NOTE: Serve this salad hot or cold.

White Fish and Vegetables en Papillote with Brown Rice

1. Preheat the oven to 325°F. Combine the onion powder, paprika, lemon pepper, red pepper flakes, garlic powder, salt, and cracked black pepper. Sprinkle over the snapper. Cut two sheets of foil larger than the fish fillets in the shape of a heart. Lightly coat the foil with cooking spray. Place a piece of fish on each piece of foil and arrange the carrots and bell pepper around the fish. Drizzle the lemon juice over the fish and vegetables and carefully seal the edges of the foil.

2. Place the packets in a shallow pan with ¼ cup water. Cover the pan and bake for 10 minutes.

To Serve: Place the packets on plates. Snip the top of the foil with scissors and let the steam escape. Serve the fish with the rice. Garnish with lemon wedges, if desired.

Servings: 2

8 ounces boneless snapper fillets

2 cups carrots cut into strips

½ cup red bell pepper cut into thin strips

2 tablespoons freshly squeezed lemon juice

1⅔ cups cooked brown rice

1 tablespoon onion powder

1 teaspoon paprika

1 teaspoon lemon pepper

1 teaspoon red pepper flakes

½ tablespoon garlic powder

Salt and cracked black pepper to taste

Cooking oil spray

Lemon wedges (optional)

Your 5-Week 5-Factor Menu Plan

These menu plans are a great way to start the 5-Factor Diet. All of the foods listed are recipes from this book. Of course, you can always make up your own menus based on the 5-Factor foods you love.

WEEK ONE

DAY 1

Breakfast: Open-Face Egg and Bacon Sandwiches, p. 121

Snack 1: Chocolate-Mint Shakes, p. 180

Lunch: Antipasto, p. 184

Snack 2: Spicy Jumbo Shrimp with Black Bean Dip, p. 156

Dinner: Southern-Style Baked Chicken with Black-Eyed Peas and Collard Greens, p. 226

DAY 2

Breakfast: Oatmeal-Berry Pancakes, p. 131

Snack 1: Hard-Boiled Eggs Stuffed with Tuna Salad, p. 152

Lunch: Green Bean Salad with Tuna and Grapefruit-Scallion Vinaigrette, p. 205

Snack 2: Chicken and Swiss Bites, p. 140

Dinner: Scallop Ratatouille, p. 221

DAY 3

Breakfast: Asparagus Crepes with Toast, p. 112

Snack 1: Apple Wedges with Cinnamon Cream, p. 174

Lunch: Snapper Ceviche with Sweet Potato Rounds, p. 204

Snack 2: Chicken Slices with Cheese and Crackers, p. 145

Dinner: Spaghetti and Meatballs, p. 228

DAY 4

Breakfast: Ham Steaks with Applesauce and Toast, p. 129

Snack 1: Sautéed Peaches with Cheese, p. 175

Lunch: Mushroom-Barley Risotto, p. 196

Snack 2: Hot Dog Skewers with Cherry Tomatoes and Pickles, p. 154

Dinner: Seared Scallops with Orange Sauce and Broccoli-Cauliflower Sauté, p. 223

DAY 5

Breakfast: Smoked Salmon Omelet with Cream Cheese and Whole Grain Toast, p. 126

Snack 1: Roasted Asparagus Spears with Turkey Slices, p. 147

Lunch: Black Bean Gumbo, p. 187

Snack 2: Berry Protein Shakes, p. 183

Dinner: Chicken Ropa Vieja, p. 211

DAY 6

Breakfast: Kashi GoLean with Nonfat Milk, p. 135

Snack 1: Roast Beef with Carrot-Pear Slaw, p. 155

Lunch: Minestrone, p. 194

Snack 2: Apple-Turkey Roll-Ups with Relish and Mustard, p. 136

Dinner: Chiles Rellenos with Brown Rice, p. 212

DAY 7

Cheat Day

WEEK TWO

DAY 1

Breakfast: Bran Pancakes with Ricotta, p. 130

Snack 1: Sautéed Apples over Rice Cakes, p. 163

Lunch: Mixed Greens with Turkey and Cheese Quesadillas, p. 195

Snack 2: Bruschetta, p. 138

Dinner: Warm White Bean, Beet, and Turkey Salad, p. 230

DAY 2

Breakfast: Fully Charged Fruit Salad, p. 133

Snack 1: Belgian Endive Stuffed with Cheesy Artichoke Spread, p. 137

Lunch: Smoked Salmon Pizza, p. 203

Snack 2: Grilled Chicken Kabobs with Carrot-Ginger Vinaigrette, p. 144

Dinner: Salmon with Cucumber-Dill Salad, p. 220

DAY 3

Breakfast: Broccoli-Cheddar Omelet, p. 117

Snack 1: Apple Wedges with Cinnamon Cream, p. 174

Lunch: Chicken and Rice Miso Soup, p. 188

Snack 2: Chips and Salsa, p. 161

Dinner: Creamy Lemon-Ginger Halibut with Corn on the Cob, p. 215

DAY 4

Breakfast: Red Bell Pepper Frittata with Baked Yams, p. 122

Snack 1: Cottage Cheese and Pears, p. 165

Lunch: Greek-Style Shrimp and Spinach Salad, p. 202

Snack 2: Crunchy Celery Sticks with Roasted-Garlic Hummus and Smoked Turkey, p. 142

Dinner: 5-Factor Lasagna, p. 208

DAY 5

Breakfast: Breakfast Burritos I, p. 114

Snack 1: Tropical Berry Protein Shakes, p. 182

Lunch: Baked Potato Skins with Sloppy Joe, p. 186

Snack 2: Gelatin with Berries and Yogurt, p. 176

Dinner: Turkey Fajitas, p. 229

DAY 6

Breakfast: Salmon-Leek Frittata with Whole Grain Toast, p. 123

Snack 1: Toast with Berries and Cocoa Cottage Cheese, p. 168

Lunch: Chicken Fingers and French Fries, p. 189

Snack 2: White Bean Dip, p. 160

Dinner: White Fish and Vegetables en Papillote with Brown Rice, p. 231

DAY 7

Cheat Day

WEEK THREE

DAY 1

Breakfast: French Toast with Ricotta, p. 132

Snack 1: Strawberry-Oatmeal Bars with Yogurt, p. 167

Lunch: Chinese Chicken Wraps with Peanut-Soy Sauce, p. 190

Snack 2: Chocolate-Berry Parfaits, p. 171

Dinner: Seared Halibut with Creamed Spinach and Brown Rice, p. 222

DAY 2

Breakfast: Sweet Potato Home Fries and Scrambled Eggs, p. 128

Snack 1: Fruit Skewers with Cottage Cheese, p. 166

Lunch: Open-Face Turkey BLT, p. 197

Snack 2: Lemon Pie, p. 179

Dinner: Country-Style Ham Steaks with Yams and Corn on the Cob, p. 213

DAY 3

Breakfast: Frittata Italiana, p. 113

Snack 1: Espresso Panna Cotta, p. 172

Lunch: Harley's Sweet Potato Melt, p. 191

Snack 2: Salmon Sashimi with Plums, p. 149

Dinner: Spaghetti and Meatballs, p. 228

DAY 4

Breakfast: Cream of Wheat and Protein, p. 134

Snack 1: Egg Salad with Toast Points, p. 150

Lunch: Baked Chicken and Black Bean Quesadillas with Salsa, p. 185

Snack 2: Fresh Figs with Balsamic Cream Sauce, p. 173

Dinner: Cream of Broccoli Soup with Sauteed Shrimp, p. 214

DAY 5

Breakfast: Scrambled Egg Casserole, p. 124

Snack 1: Chocolate-Mint Shakes, p. 180

Lunch: Pink Pizza, p. 198

Snack 2: Smoked Turkey and Fruit Salad, p. 148

Dinner: Crispy Chicken Tostada, p. 216

DAY 6

Breakfast: Egg and Veggie Muffins, p. 120

Snack 1: Spinach Frittata and Toast, p. 153

Lunch: Salmon Tartare with Arugula, p. 201

Snack 2: Chicken and Swiss Bites, p. 140

Dinner: Bison Steak with Cauliflower-Carrot Mash and Brown Rice, p. 217

DAY 7

Cheat Day

WEEK FOUR

DAY 1

Breakfast: Ham Steaks with Applesauce and Toast., p. 129

Snack 1: Berry Protein Shakes, p. 183

Lunch: Salad Niçoise, p. 200

Snack 2: Egg and Celery Platter with Mustard-Balsamic Sauce, p. 151

Dinner: Indian-Style Chicken with Curried Yogurt Sauce and Brown Rice, p. 218

DAY 2

Breakfast: Oatmeal-Berry Pancakes, p. 131

Snack 1: Apple-Turkey Roll-Ups with Relish and Mustard, p. 136

Lunch: Stuffed Mushrooms and Greens, p. 206

Snack 2: Chicken Salad with Apples, p. 141

Dinner: Lobster and Peas with Tomato-Basil Sauce and Barley, p. 219

DAY 3

Breakfast: Scrambled Eggs with Toast and Grapefruit, p. 125

Snack 1: Raspberry Gelatin with Cottage Cheese, p. 177

Lunch: Mixed Greens with Turkey and Cheese Quesadillas, p. 195

Snack 2: Edamame and Tuna Sashimi with Ginger-Scallion Vinaigrette, p. 143

Dinner: Shrimp and Rice Stir-Fry, p. 225

DAY 4

Breakfast: Breakfast Burritos II, p. 115

Snack 1: Carrot Sticks with Onion Dip, p. 151

Lunch: Antipasto, p. 184

Snack 2: Cheese Course, p. 139

Dinner: Southern-Style Baked Chicken with Black-Eyed Peas and Collard Greens, p. 226

DAY 5

Breakfast: Smoked Turkey and Tomato Scrambled Eggs with Toast, p. 127

Snack 1: Pesto Crisps with Tomatoes and Cheese, p. 162

Lunch: Minestrone, p. 194

Snack 2: Cheesecake, p. 170

Dinner: Salmon with Cucumber-Dill Salad, p. 220

DAY 6

Breakfast: Bell Pepper Pancakes with Mozzarella and Crisp Bacon, p. 118

Snack 1: Pears with Peanut Butter Dip, p. 164

Lunch: Mediterranean-Style Chicken and Quinoa Salad, p. 192

Snack 2: Chips and Salsa, p. 161

Dinner: Chicken Chow Mein, p. 210

DAY 7

Cheat Day

WEEK FIVE

DAY 1

Breakfast: Smoked Salmon Omelet with Cream Cheese and Whole Grain Toast, p. 126

Snack 1: Sauteed Apples over Rice Cakes, p. 163

Lunch: Black Bean Gumbo, p. 187

Snack 2: Crunchy Celery Sticks with Roasted-Garlic Hummus and Smoked Turkey, p. 142

Dinner: 5-Factor Lasagna, p. 208

DAY 2

Breakfast: Open-Face Egg and Bacon Sandwiches, p. 121

Snack 1: Pear and Arugula Salad with Ricotta, p. 146

Lunch: Tuscan Tomato Soup, p. 207

Snack 2: Chicken Slices with Cheese and Crackers, p. 145

Dinner: Argentine-Style Steak Salad with Watercress and Mustard-Cilantro Vinaigrette, p. 209

DAY 3

Breakfast: The Cowboy Omelet, p. 119

Snack 1: Passion Fruit and Tangerine Shakes, p. 181

Lunch: Mexican Chicken Salad with Spicy Salsa Dressing, p. 193

Snack 2: Bruschetta, p. 138

Dinner: Shrimp and Tofu Soup, p. 224

DAY 4

Breakfast: Breakfast Burritos III, p. 116

Snack 1: Toast with Berries and Cocoa Cottage Cheese, p. 168

Lunch: Mixed Greens with Turkey and Cheese Quesadillas, p. 195

Snack 2: Butterscotch and Apple Pudding, p. 169

Dinner: Chicken Ropa Vieja, p. 211

DAY 5

Breakfast: Asparagus Crepes with Toast, p. 112

Snack 1: Grilled Chicken Kabobs with Carrot-Ginger Vinaigrette, p. 144

Lunch: Mushroom Barley Risotto, p. 196

Snack 2: Berry Protein Shakes, p. 183

Dinner: Scallop Ratatouille, p. 221

DAY 6

Breakfast: Broccoli-Cheddar Omelet, p. 117

Snack 1: Fruit Skewers with Cottage Cheese, p. 166

Lunch: Portobello and Turkey Stacks, p. 199

Snack 2: Lemon Yogurt with Kiwi, p. 178

Dinner: Soy-Poached Chicken with Vegetables and Brown Rice, p. 227

DAY 7

Cheat Day

CHAPTER 11

5-Factor Success Log

Writing down what you eat makes you think about your food three times.

First, you think about it as you eat it.

Second, you think about it when you write it down.

Third, you think about it when you read later on.

I've found that thinking three times about everything you eat gives you a sense of ownership of your actions. It also gives you a mini-assessment every day on how well you're doing with your diet. Rome wasn't built in one night. Seeing a few weeks' worth of food logs that show how much better you're eating can be the inspiration you need to stay the course. In fact it's been shown that people who keep track of what they eat are more successful with their nutritional goals.

Still I know you don't have time to write down every calorie and every fat gram from every bite you eat. I wouldn't expect that from my clients, and I don't expect it from you. So here's the good news: You don't have to.

Keeping track of how well you're doing on the 5-Factor Diet isn't painful. It doesn't require a calculator or more than a few seconds of your time.

All of the recipes in this book incorporate 5-Factor Diet requirements—you don't even have to think about them.

When you're ready to create your own meals and daily menus based on the 5-Factor principles—and using the 5-Factor Must-Have Foods—this easy-to-use chart will help you track your progress. (Make copies of it to use every day.)

Record the three foods—a low-fat protein, a low- to moderate-GI carb, and a no- to low-sugar beverage—you plan to eat at each of the five meals of the day. As for the fiber column, if you're eating a low-GI carb, I guarantee it contains the 5 to 10 grams of fiber required at each meal. If necessary, add another fibrous carbohydrate—beans or spinach, for example—to your meal so you can write "yes" in the fiber column. You must have 5 to 10 grams of fiber at every meal to follow the 5-Factor Diet.

The last column, healthy fats, needn't read "yes" at every meal. Just be sure you aren't eating any unhealthy saturated or trans fats.

Ready to start your 5-Factor day? Here you go!

5-FACTOR DIET DAY—SAMPLE

Here's what an average day of eating on the 5-Factor Diet might look like:

Meal	Protein	Low- to moderate-GI carbs	No- to low-sugar beverage	Does it have 5–10 grams of fiber?	Does it have healthy fats? *
Breakfast	3 egg whites	Food for Life's Ezekiel No-Flour Cinnamon Bread toast	Coffee with Splenda	Yes	Yes
Snack I	Fat-free cheese slice	I-2 apples	Diet soda	Yes	Yes
Lunch	Chicken sandwich w/mustard; side of black beans	Food for Life's Ezekiel No-Flour Tortilla Wrap	Diet Snapple	Yes	Yes
Snack 2	Turkey jerky	Side of steamed veggies	Sugar-free Hansen's	Yes	Yes
Dinner	Steamed salmon	Kashi 7 Whole Grain Pilaf	Green tea	Yes	Yes

*Note: Not every meal must include a healthy fat. For instance, you may choose a low- or no-fat snack that still fits the rest of the 5-Factor criteria. Just be sure that your meal does not include any unhealthy fats (saturated fats or trans fats).

YOUR 5-FACTOR DIET DAY

Meal	Protein	Low- to moderate- GI carbs	No- to low-sugar beverage	Does it have 5–10 grams of fiber?	Does it have healthy fats?*
Breakfast					
Snack 1					
Lunch					
Snack 2					
Dinner					

*Note: Not every meal must include a healthy fat. For instance, you may choose a low- or no-fat snack that still fits the rest of the 5-Factor criteria. Just be sure that your meal does not include any unhealthy fats (saturated fats or trans fats).

YOUR 5-FACTOR DIET DAY

Meal	Protein	Low- to moderate- GI carbs	No- to low-sugar beverage	Does it have 5–10 grams of fiber?	Does it have healthy fats?*
Breakfast					
Snack I					
Lunch					
Snack 2					
Dinner					

*Note: Not every meal must include a healthy fat. For instance, you may choose a low- or no-fat snack that still fits the rest of the 5-Factor criteria. Just be sure that your meal does not include any unhealthy fats (saturated fats or trans fats).

YOUR 5-FACTOR WEEKLY PLAN

Once you get used to designing your 5-Factor meals, it's easy to design your own weekly meal plan, using many of the foods I suggested earlier—especially the 5-Factor Must-Have Foods.

YOUR 5-FACTOR DIET WEEK

Meal	Breakfast	Snack I	Lunch	Snack 2	Dinner
Monday					
Tuesday					
Wednesday					
Thursday					
Friday					
Saturday					
Sunday	Cheat Day!				

YOUR 5-FACTOR DIET WEEK

Meal	Breakfast	Snack I	Lunch	Snack 2	Dinner
Monday					
Tuesday					
Wednesday					
Thursday					
Friday					
Saturday					
Sunday	Cheat Day!				

Index

Recipe Index